Manual of
Laboratory Tests for Nurses

Manual of
Laboratory Tests for Nurses

Ramnik Sood
MBBS, PGEn&OH, MD (Pathology, Gold Medallist)
Director
Speciality Diagnostic Labs
Panjim, Goa, India

Consultant Pathologist/Cyto-Histopathologist
RMDC, AVIVO Group, UAE

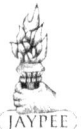

JAYPEE BROTHERS MEDICAL PUBLISHERS
The Health Sciences Publisher
New Delhi | London

Jaypee Brothers Medical Publishers (P) Ltd

Headquarters

Jaypee Brothers Medical Publishers (P) Ltd
EMCA House, 23/23-B
Ansari Road, Daryaganj
New Delhi 110 002, India
Landline: +91-11-23272143, +91-11-23272703
+91-11-23282021, +91-11-23245672
Email: jaypee@jaypeebrothers.com

Corporate Office

Jaypee Brothers Medical Publishers (P) Ltd
4838/24, Ansari Road, Daryaganj
New Delhi 110 002, India
Phone: +91-11-43574357
Fax: +91-11-43574314
Email: jaypee@jaypeebrothers.com

Overseas Office

J.P. Medical Ltd
83 Victoria Street, London
SW1H 0HW (UK)
Phone: +44 20 3170 8910
Fax: +44 (0)20 3008 6180
Email: info@jpmedpub.com

Website: www.jaypeebrothers.com
Website: www.jaypeedigital.com

© 2022, Jaypee Brothers Medical Publishers

The views and opinions expressed in this book are solely those of the original contributor(s)/author(s) and do not necessarily represent those of editor(s) of the book.

All rights reserved. No part of this publication may be reproduced, stored or transmitted in any form or by any means, electronic, mechanical, photocopying, recording or otherwise, without the prior permission in writing of the publishers.

All brand names and product names used in this book are trade names, service marks, trademarks or registered trademarks of their respective owners. The publisher is not associated with any product or vendor mentioned in this book.

Medical knowledge and practice change constantly. This book is designed to provide accurate, authoritative information about the subject matter in question. However, readers are advised to check the most current information available on procedures included and check information from the manufacturer of each product to be administered, to verify the recommended dose, formula, method and duration of administration, adverse effects and contraindications. It is the responsibility of the practitioner to take all appropriate safety precautions. Neither the publisher nor the author(s)/editor(s) assume any liability for any injury and/or damage to persons or property arising from or related to use of material in this book.

This book is sold on the understanding that the publisher is not engaged in providing professional medical services. If such advice or services are required, the services of a competent medical professional should be sought.

Every effort has been made where necessary to contact holders of copyright to obtain permission to reproduce copyright material. If any have been inadvertently overlooked, the publisher will be pleased to make the necessary arrangements at the first opportunity.

Inquiries for bulk sales may be solicited at: jaypee@jaypeebrothers.com

Manual of Laboratory Tests for Nurses

First Edition: **2022**

ISBN: 978-93-5465-574-6

Preface

In clinical practice nursing staff is not always in contact with the clinician/consultant and has to sometimes take minor decisions in emergency situations.

This book outlines and highlights the laboratory investigations and the related normal values (both in conventional and SI units). It gives what to make of physical features of body excreta, e.g., urine, stool, CSF, gastric fluids, sputum, etc.

It also gives how to obtain/process samples for submission to a clinical laboratory. Simple points of care tests like Uristix, etc., are also explained in ample detail for quick understanding.

If you are a budding Florence Nightingale or already an established one, you shall find this book very handy in your day-to-day work.

Happy reading and learning!

Ramnik Sood

Contents

1. **Common Abbreviations Used in Laboratory Investigations** 1
   - Conventional Units *1*
   - SI Units (International System of Units) *2*

2. **Introduction** 3
   - The Probabilistic Nature of Diagnosis *3*
   - Purposes for Ordering Laboratory Tests *4*
   - Diagnosis *4*
   - Monitoring Therapy *4*
   - Screening *4*

3. **Sample Collection by Technical Personnel and Ward Sisters** 5
   - Procedure of Sample Collection *6*
   - Procedure of Venipuncture *8*
   - Order of Draw *8*
   - Sample Collection Order Form/Requisition *11*
   - Procedural Issues *12*
   - Performance of Fingerstick Collection *15*
   - Other Collection Issues *16*
   - Safety and Infection Control *19*
   - Troubleshooting Guidelines *20*
   - Blood Sampling System *24*

4. SI Units and Conversion Tables 25
- Litre *25*
- Gram *27*
- Mole (Mol) *27*
- International Unit (U) *28*
- Conversion Factors between Conventional and System International Units (SIU) *28*

5. Body Excreta Analysis 48
Urine Analysis 48
- Composition of Urine *48*
- Gross Examination of Urine *51*
- Multiple® Reagent Strips for Urinalysis *61*

Stool Examination 79

6. Body Fluids Analysis 89
Cerebrospinal and other Body Fluids 89
- Cerebrospinal Fluid *89*
- Pleural Fluid *92*
- Pericardial Fluid (PF) *95*
- Peritoneal Fluid *95*
- Amniocentesis and Amniotic Fluid Analysis, Diagnostic *98*

7. Sputum Examination 101
- Specimen Collection *101*
- Sputum Examination *102*

8. Laboratory Investigations 105
- Hematology *105*
- Serum, Plasma and Whole Blood Chemistries *108*
- Urine Chemistry *122*
- Immunodiagnostic Test *128*
- Cerebrospinal Fluid *131*
- Miscellaneous Values *132*

9. Profile of Laboratory Tests According to Body Systems 138
- Cardiovascular System *138*
- Pulmonary System *143*
- Neurological System *145*
- Hematological System *148*
- Endocrine System *154*
- Renal and Urologic System *160*
- Musculoskeletal System *164*
- Hepatobiliary–GI Systems *168*
- Reproductive System *174*
- Immune and Autoimmune Conditions *181*
- Tumors *184*

Index 187

Chapter 1
Common Abbreviations Used in Laboratory Investigations

CONVENTIONAL UNITS

Kg	=	Kilogram
gm	=	gram
mg	=	milligram
µg	=	microgram
µµg	=	micromicrogram
ng	=	nanogram
pg	=	picogram
dl	=	decilitre
ml	=	millilitre
cu. mm	=	cubic millimetre
fL	=	femtolitre
mM	=	millimole
nM	=	nanomole
mOsm	=	milliosmole
mm	=	millimetre
µm	=	micron or micrometre
U	=	unit
mU	=	milliunit
µU	=	microunit

mEq = milliequivalent
IU = International Unit
mIU = milli-international Unit
mm Hg = millimetres of mercury

SI UNITS (INTERNATIONAL SYSTEM OF UNITS)

gm = gram
L = litre
d = day
h = hour
mol = mole
mmol = millimole
μmol = micromole
nmol = nanomole
pmol = picomole.

Chapter 2

Introduction

The term diagnostic test does not refer only to costly tests imaging or monitoring procedures like MRI, CT or cardiac catheterization. It refers in addition to the countless laboratory tests ordered everyday on patients such as electrolytes, serum chemistries, coagulation profiles or blood counts.

Understanding laboratory investigations provides nurses with essential and easily digested information about the most frequently requested tests that are performed on patients. It explains the physiological function being measured, details of reference ranges and clinical significance of test results for diagnosis or patient monitoring. Test results that warrant immediate clinical intervention are identified and wherever possible, abnormal test results are related to symptoms.

THE PROBABILISTIC NATURE OF DIAGNOSIS

Diagnosis is an uncertain art. This remains true in early phases of diagnostic evaluation. Studies of physicians reasoning have demonstrated that, as physician evaluate patients they keep a limited set of five to seven diagnostic hypotheses in mind, each of which is assigned, a relative probability such as 'very likely', 'possible', or 'unlikely'. These relative probabilities are adjusted upward or downward depending new information gained through history, physical examination and diagnostic tests. With enough information one diagnostic possibility becomes likely enough for the physicians to stop further investigations and declare that possibility as 'diagnosis'.

PURPOSES FOR ORDERING LABORATORY TESTS

The purposes for which tests are obtained have a great deal to do with both the choice of diagnostic tests and its interpretation. One survey of physicians in a large teaching hospital found that three general reasons accounted for most laboratory tests ordering: Diagnosis (37%), monitoring therapy (33%) and screening for asymptomatic disease (32%).

DIAGNOSIS

In order to use a test for diagnostic purposes, the test has to be positive in a large proportion of patients with disease—high sensitivity and negative in a large proportion without the disease—high specificity. Ideally, for the test to be maximally useful for diagnostic use, both sensitivity and specificity should be 100%.

MONITORING THERAPY

Whenever a test is repeated in order to follow a therapeutic drug level or observe for side effects, it is being used for monitoring purposes.

SCREENING

The object of the use of diagnostic tests for screening is to detect diseases in its earliest, presymptomatic state when, presumably, it is less widespread and more easily treated or cured. Most screening programs, such as occult blood screening or mammography are aimed at cancer detection.

Chapter 3

Sample Collection by Technical Personnel and Ward Sisters

INTRODUCTION

Collections of sample of blood, urine, stool, swabs and a few other procedures are routinely performed in the Hospital settings as well as outside **(Table 3.1)**. The purpose of this chapter is to know about the procedure of sample collection, about the policies, standard operating procedure, proper safety, maintenance of time and understanding the nature of urgency.

Policy

This varies in every set up according to the decision of the management. However, a few are commonly thought about, discussed and finally implemented. The policies of sample collection in hospital set up are following:

Table 3.1: List of samples in hospital setup.

- Venous blood
- Capillary blood
- Arterial puncture
- Urine collection directly or from urobags
- Stool
- Swabs, etc.

- Proper collection of sample by trained personnel.
- Maintenance of time in all respects.
- Maintenance of safety measures in routine and regular fashion as well as in emergency situations.
- Counseling.
- Adequate communication with the information system.

PROCEDURE OF SAMPLE COLLECTION

Collection of peripheral venous blood is known as Phlebotomy and personnel who are trained for this are known as Phlebotomists. Ward sisters are usually trained enough for that.

The nature of sample, the specificity of the tests, time of collections are all done according to the directions of the attending medical personnel. Collection of samples other than blood are also performed in the same way.

Largely phlebotomies are done while the patient is lying on the bed, awake, properly introduced. A short while procedure of counseling of the patient in assertive manner to avoid panic and to reduce pain.

Gentleness, patience, knowledge and purpose of the activity are of prime importance to win the confidence of the ailing. For conscious inquisitive patients care must be taken to answer their queries.

Selection of the site venipuncture is the next matter to be thought. Antecubital veins are most preferred sites. Other sites are forearm, dorsum of wrist, neck, sides of the heel and femoral veins.

The limb should be free from infusion or transfusion set up. In cases when both upper limbs even all four limbs are occupied with fluid lines or channels, one can find veins in the neck. In small babies skin puncture at inferolateral or inferomedial aspects of the heel can also be used with similar yield.

Situations where no favorable sites are available for venipuncture, one can stop on infusion set, wait for a few minutes and draw blood sample. Selection of vein is state of art. Subcutaneous veins are better seen than felt. Skin fairness facilitates this issue. However, experienced personnel with sensitive finger tips, focus and concentration can feel the veins easily in any kind of situations. A good eyesight is mandatory.

Sample collection trolley is to be made available before everything. A collection tray should have the following in order to have a smooth function of the procedure **(Table 3.2)**.

Table 3.2: Instruments for collection tray.

- Sterile and disposable nitrile gloves
- Large achromatic eye covering goggles
- Pared nails to facilitate palpation and to avoid injuries
- Adequate syringes with proper needles or evacuated vials with holders and special double ended needles
- Sterile swabs with 70% isopropanol in water
- Tube stand
- Tourniquet
- Stop watch
- Glass capillaries
- Round filter paper
- Thermometer and pulse oximeter, if necessary
- Receptacles for disposal of the waste
- Clean glass slide and a good spreader for smearing
- Pencil, glass marking pen and diamond marker
- Betadine
- Tissue paper

PROCEDURE OF VENIPUNCTURE

A rubber tourniquet or an elastic arm tourniquet is tied a few centimetres above the chosen site. Tourniquet can be tied for a period <1 minute duration. It is not wise to waste time for cleaning the puncture site after applying the tourniquet. A small straight segment (at least of > 2 cm long) of a palpable vein is fixed and made prominent by grabbing the elbow from behind and asking the patient to clench the fist. The needle should be introduced gently, in a straight or swing fashion at an angle of 15° to 30° from the skin surface within seconds into the lumen of the desired vein. Blood is immediately seen at the base of the needle when hypodermic syringe is used. However, it is totally blind in case of evacuated system of collection. In the former, a fixed volume of blood can be drawn by a single puncture. On the other hand, multiple vials can be filled in case of evacuated sampling. However, one can use butterfly needle for any volume of blood.

Once the vein is punctured tourniquet and the clenched fist are to be released immediately. In cases of collections of blood for calcium and lithium both tourniquet and clenching must not be done.

Glove hygiene is to be maintained in every individual patient. The personnel are to clean hands before and after use of single set of gloves. Needlestick should be avoided by all means.

ORDER OF DRAW

A definite order is maintained to avoid cross contamination of additives between the tubes **(Table 3.3)**. The order of sampling is as follows.

- **1st:** Blood culture in bottle or yellow/black topped plastic tube containing broth mixture. The latter keeps the viability of the microorganisms and make it suitable for cultures of aerobes, anaerobes and fungi.

Table 3.3: Vacutainer/sample tube types for venipuncture/phlebotomy.

Tube cap color or type	Additive	Usage and comments
Blood culture bottle	Sodium polyanethol sulfonate (anticoagulant) and growth media for microorganisms	Usually drawn first for minimal risk of contamination. Two bottles are typically collected in one blood draw; one for aerobic organisms and one for anaerobic organisms
Light blue	Sodium citrate (anticoagulant)	Coagulation tests such as prothrombin time (PT) and partial thromboplastin time (PTT) and thrombin time (TT). Tube must be filled 100%
Plain red	No additive	Serum: Total complement activity, cryoglobulins
Gold	Clot activator and serum separating gel	Serum-separating tube: Tube inversions promote clotting. Most chemistry, endocrine and serology tests, including hepatitis and HIV
Dark green	Sodium heparin (anticoagulant)	Chromosome testing, HLA typing, ammonia, lactate
Mint green	Lithium heparin (anticoagulant)	Plasma. Tube inversions prevent clotting
Lavender (purple)	EDTA (chelator/anticoagulant)	Whole blood: CBC, ESR, Coombs test, platelet antibodies, flow cytometry, blood levels of tacrolimus and cyclosporin

Contd...

Contd...

Tube cap color or type	Additive	Usage and comments
Pink	EDTA (chelator/anticoagulant)	Blood typing and cross-matching, direct Coombs test, HIV viral load
Royal blue	EDTA (chelator/anticoagulant)	Trace elements, heavy metals, most drug levels, toxicology
Tan	EDTA (chelator/anticoagulant)	Lead
Gray	• Sodium fluoride (glycolysis inhibitor) • Potassium oxalate (anticoagulant)	Glucose, lactate
Yellow	Acid-citrate-dextrose A (anticoagulant)	Tissue typing, DNA studies, HIV cultures
Pearl (white)	Separating gel and (K_2) EDTA	PCR for adenovirus, toxoplasma and HHV-6

- **2nd:** Coagulation tube for routine coagulation assay if ordered only. If there is a concern about tissue thromboplastin, then one may draw a non-additive tube first and light blue topped coagulation tube containing Na-citrate. In this case blood is to be drawn upto the mark.
- **3rd:** Red topped non-additive tubes are used next for Chemistries, Immunology, Serology and Blood bank purposes.
- **4th:** Afterwards all tubes containing additives are used in the following order. The SST (Serum separation tube) containing a

gel separates serum (top) and blood (bottom) on centrifugation. These tubes are gold capped.
- **5th:** Orange topped tube containing thrombin which quickly clots blood and express serum quickly. This is used for urgent situations.
- **6th:** Light green lithium heparin tube with plasma gel separating tube (PST) for chemistries.
- **7th:** Dark green topped Na-heparin anticoagulant tube for chromosome testings, HLA typing, ammonia and lactate estimations.
- **8th:** Lavender or purple topped tube with EDTA as additive for complete blood count, ESR, Blood bank. This requires full draw and proper mixing. Other uses are: Direct Coombs test, Platelet antibodies, Flow cytometries, Blood level of tacrolimus, Cyclosporine.

Each sample container is to be labelled for proper identification immediately after the sample collection. The label should contain patient's name, test name, time. A bar code sticker can be pasted for better information.

SAMPLE COLLECTION ORDER FORM/REQUISITION

A requisition form must accompany each sample submitted to the laboratory. This order form must be in duplicate and must accompany individual's samples in zipped plastic bag to the lab. The following are the essential elements of an order form:
- Patient's name, age, sex.
- Patient's ID: Hospital ID and a personal ID.
- Date of birth.
- Doctor's name and telephone number.
- Date and time of the order.

- Date and time of collection.
- Collector's name and signature.
- Primary samples, e.g., blood, urine, etc.
- Tests required.

PROCEDURAL ISSUES

- The sample collector must apply a complete professional and courteous attitude to gain the confidence of the patient and be satisfied with the whole process.
- Greet the patient at the same time the collector clears his/her identification to the patient. Express in brief about the purpose and procedure confidently and gently. Both verbal and nonverbal communications are essential. If possible speak with the patient during the procedure to keep the patient's attention away. Always thank the patient and excuse yourself courteously when the procedure is completed.

Patient's Bill of Rights

The patient has the right to:
- Impartial access to treatment or accommodations that are available or medically indicated, regardless of race, creed, sex, national origin, or sources of payment for care.
- Considerate and respectful care.
- Confidentiality of all communications and other records pertaining to the patient's care.
- Expect that any discussion or consultation involving the patient's case will be conducted discretely and that individuals not directly involved in the case will not be present without patient permission.
- Expect reasonable safety congruent with the hospital practices and environment.

- Know the identity and professional status of individuals providing service and to know which physician or other practitioner is primarily responsible for his or her care.
- Obtain from the practitioner complete and current information about diagnosis, treatment, and any known prognosis, in terms the patient can reasonably be expected to understand.
- Reasonable informed participation in decisions involving the patient's health care. The patient shall be informed if the hospital proposes to engage in or perform human experimentation or other research/educational profits affecting his or her care or treatment. The patient has the right to refuse participation in such activity.
- Consult a specialist at the patient's own request and expense.
- Refuse treatment to the extent permitted by law.
- Regardless of the source of payment, request and receive an itemized and detailed explanation of the total bill for services rendered in the hospital.
- Be informed of the hospital rules and regulations regarding patient conduct.

Issues on Venipuncture Site Selection

Although the median cubital vein or cephalic vein of the arm are most commonly selected for venipuncture, other veins like basilic vein, veins of dorsum of arm, veins of dorsum of wrist may used. However, foot veins are least commonly used as chances of complications are more common.

Sites to be Avoided for Venipuncture
- Foot veins
- Scar over burns or surgery

- Upper extremities on the side of mastectomy as the results of the tests may be affected by lymphedema.
- Avoid hematoma to get rid of erroneous results.
- Intravenous line in one arm: One can use the arm or the same as distal to the IV line puncture site. In the case of the latter, it is advisable to turn of the flow of the IV line for at least 2 minutes before the sample collection. Apply the tourniquet below the IV site, avoid the same vein being used for the infusion line; draw and discard at least 5 ml of blood and finally draw for tests.
- Drawing from the IV line may be rarely needed but warrant problems. However, one has to flush the line first. Then using butterfly needle, one has to discard at 5 ml of blood before using for tests.
- Cannula: Drawing blood from cannula or fistula with heparin lock should not be done without consulting the attending physician.

Palpation of Vein is an Art

- Veins are soft compressible without any pulsation. Vein can rolled under the palpating fingertips.
- Verify the following details about the patient's condition before phlebotomy, such as state of fasting and its duration, dietary restrictions, medications, history of allergies to antiseptics or adhesives.
- Patient's position is important to get the most suitable site of venipuncture. Arm should be hyperextended.
- The tourniquet is to be placed at least 3–4 inches above the chosen site of venipuncture. The tourniquet is never to be kept tight for more than two minutes. If so, one has to release it immediately, wait for another two minutes and then reapply.

- Prepare the patient's arm using an alcohol prep. Cleanse in a circular fashion, beginning at the site and working outward. Allow to dry.
- Patient should be asked to clench the fist without pumping.
- The needle should angle 15° to 30° to the surface. Needle is to be inserted steadily without trauma and excessive probing.
- When the last tube to be drawn is filling, remove the tourniquet.
- While withdrawing the needle, press the gauze deeper and after complete withdrawal of the needle press the gauze tightly.
- Mix and label all the tubes and place within a zipped plastic bag.
- Dispose all the contaminated materials to the designated containers.

PERFORMANCE OF FINGERSTICK COLLECTION

The best locations for fingersticks are the 3rd (middle) and 4th (ring) fingers of the non-dominant hand. Do not use the tip of the finger or the center of the finger. Avoid the side of the finger where there is less soft tissue, where vessels and nerves are located, and where the bone is closer to the surface. The 2nd (index) finger tends to have thicker, callused skin. The fifth finger tends to have less soft tissue overlying the bone. Avoid puncturing a finger that is cold or cyanotic, swollen, scarred, or covered with a rash.

- Using a sterile lancet, make a skin puncture just off the center of the finger pad. The puncture should be made perpendicular to the ridges of the fingerprint so that the drop of blood does not run down the ridges.
- Wipe away the first drop of blood, which tends to contain excess tissue fluid.
- Collect drops of blood into the collection device by gently massaging the finger. Avoid excessive pressure that may squeeze tissue fluid into the drop of blood.

- Cap, rotate and invert the collection device to mix the blood collected.
- Have the patient hold a small gauze pad over the puncture site for a couple of minutes to stop the bleeding.
- Dispose of contaminated materials/supplies in designated containers.
- Label all appropriate tubes at the patient bedside.
- Deliver specimens promptly to the laboratory.

OTHER COLLECTION ISSUES

Prevention of Hematoma

- Complete penetration of the superficial wall of the major superficial vein and continue penetration for a certain distain distance show that the needle tip remains within the venous lumen sufficiently and safely inside; never to penetrate through the deeper wall of the vein. Both partial penetration and penetration of both the walls lead to hematoma.
- To keep a continuous pressure on the puncture site by the other hand till the needle is removed.
- Always remove the tourniquet before removal of the needle.
- Put firm pressure at the puncture site after removal of the needle.

Prevention of Hemolysis

- Always mix blood with its anticoagulant gently, thoroughly, continuously and completely (5-10 times).
- In case of hypodermic syringe and needle, the needle should not be too thin, the plunger of the syringe should not be drawn out forcefully and suddenly, there should not be any creation of froth or bubbles within the syringe.

- Never to draw blood from a hematoma.
- The venipuncture site should be dry.
- Avoid too much probing or negotiation to get the venous wall or its lumen.
- Avoid prolonged application of tourniquet or clenching of patient's fist.

Indwelling Catheter

- Avoid it as it contains heparin to keep the catheter patent. This is a potential source of error.
- To avoid the error one has to discard at least a few ml of blood before actually filling the collection tubes.

Prevention of Hemoconcentration

In this situation there is an increase in concentration of larger molecules. To prevent that one has to take care of the following:
- Never to keep the tourniquet fastened and tight for more than 1 minute (vide infra).
- Never to ask the patient to keep the fist clenched once the drawing of blood is started.
- Never to ask the patient to pump by the fist during the time of drawing of blood.
- Not to massage or probe the puncture site.
- Not to use indwelling catheter, prolonged used for infusion, sclerosed or thrombosed veins.

Prolonged Tourniquet Application

- This leads to increase in local increase of hydrostatic pressure → passage of water and filterable elements out of the blood vessels → hemoconcentration.

- Hemoconcentration leads to increase in serum total protein, AST, total lipids, cholesterol, iron, etc. There may be increase in Hct, and other cellular parameters of blood.
- Prolonged tourniquet application leads to hemolysis and erroneous increase in serum potassium.

Patient Preparation Factors

- Maintain proper time of collecting samples
- Patient should be away from exhaustive activities before sampling. Patient should preferably remain restful for at 10–15 minnutes before sample collection procedures. Exercise leads to increase in creatine kinase (CK), lactate dehydrogenase (LDH), aspartate aminotransferase (AST) and platelet count.

Therapeutic Drug Monitoring

Different pharmacologic agents have patterns of administration, body distribution, metabolism, and elimination that affect the drug concentration as measured in the blood. Many drugs will have "peak" and "trough" levels that vary according to dosage levels and intervals. Check for timing instructions for drawing the appropriate samples.

Diurnal Rhythm

Diurnal rhythm is an important factor in cases of serum cortisol which is highest in the morning and go to its nadir in the afternoon. Serum iron remains low during daytime than during the dusk.

Posture is an important factor in cases of large filterable materials in blood. Enzymes, proteins, lipids, iron, and calcium are significantly increased with changes in position.

Other Factors

Age, sex or pregnancy may affect the test results. The reference values are to be written as per age, sex or other state matched.

Reasons for Cancellation of Tests

- Nontechnical reasons:
    - Duplicate test request
    - Incorrect test ordered
    - Test no longer needed
- Technical reasons:
    - Hemolysis of the specimen
    - Clotted specimen
    - Quantity of specimen not sufficient
    - Collection of specimen in incorrect tube
    - Contaminated specimen
    - Identification of the specimen is suspected
    - Delay in transport – specimen too old.

SAFETY AND INFECTION CONTROL

Protect Yourself

- Because the ward sisters or hospital lab collectors are almost always with the patients, knowledge of protecting oneself about prevention from infection, accident or infections are to be kept in mind.
- Protections: Wearing gloves, lab coats, eye shield with regular and judicious changing of gloves, washing hands after each set of collection.
- Dispose of items in appropriate containers.

- Dispose of needles immediately upon removal from the patient's vein. Do not bend, break, recap, or re-sheath needles to avoid accidental needle puncture or splashing of contents.
- Clean up any blood spills with a disinfectant such as freshly made 2% bleach.

Measures in cases of accidental stick by contaminated needle:
- Remove the gloves and dispose of them properly.
- Squeeze puncture site to promote bleeding.
- Wash the area well with soap and water.
- Record the patient's name and ID number.
- Follow institution's guidelines regarding treatment and follow-up.

Protect the Patient

- Place the collection material and collected samples away from the patients especially suffering from psychiatric illness or children.
- Maintain cleanliness and prevent cross contamination.

TROUBLESHOOTING GUIDELINES

If there is an Incomplete Collection or No Blood is Obtained

The following are a few measures:
- Change the position of the needle. Move it forward (it may not be in the lumen) or move it backward (it may have penetrated too far).
- Adjust the angle (the bevel may be against the vein wall).
- Loosen the tourniquet. It may be obstructing blood flow.

- Try another tube. Use a smaller tube with less vacuum. There may be no vacuum in the tube being used.
- Re-anchor the vein. Veins sometimes roll away from the point of the needle and puncture site.
- Have the patient make a fist and flex the arm, which helps engorge muscles to fill veins.
- Pre-warm the region of the vein to reduce vasoconstriction and increase blood flow.
- Have the patient drink fluids if dehydrated.

If Blood Stops Flowing into the Tube or Syringe

- Re-secure the tourniquet to increase the venous pressure. If that is not successful then withdraw the needle, take care of the puncture site and choose another puncture site for a repeat puncture.
- Hold the collecting needle holder firmly against the skin to vein junction to keep the needle tip in position.

Other Troubleshootings

Inadvertent puncture of artery: Blood is usually bright red. The puncture site is to be secured very firmly for a prolonged period.

If hematoma is already formed, stop collection, withdraw the needle, secure the puncture site till there is no increase in the size of hematoma. Consult attending physician for further management of the hematoma.

Blood Collections on Babies

Inferolateral and inferomedial aspect of the pre-warmed (at 42°C) heel are sites of collection of newborn babies blood. Take meticulous care about the pre-warming temperature. Hold the baby steadily and firmly. Clean the area with alcohol sponge and dry it with sterile cotton pad. Using sterile lancet cut the sides of the heel so that a clear drop of blood comes out immediately. Wipe away the first drop of blood with sterile dry cotton.

- Fill the capillary tube(s) or micro collection device(s) as needed.
- When finished, elevate the heel, place a piece of clean, dry cotton on the puncture site, and hold it in place until the bleeding has stopped.
- Be sure to dispose of the lancet in the appropriate sharps container.
- Dispose of contaminated materials in appropriate waste receptacles.
- Remove your gloves and wash your hands.

Pediatric Phlebotomy

Children, particularly under the age of 10, may experience pain and anxiety during the phlebotomy procedure. A variety of techniques can be employed to reduce pain and anxiety. Effective methods use distraction. These may include listening to music or a story, watching a video, playing with a toy, having a parent provide distraction with talk or touch, using flash cards, and squeezing a rubber ball.

Femoral puncture is an age old procedure for collection of blood. With appropriate hand this is done quite smoothly. However, the risk of femoral arterial puncture is high and the method is not very attractive now-a-days.

Collection Tubes for Phlebotomy

- Collection tubes can vary in size for volume of blood drawn, appropriate to the tests ordered with sample size required, and

vary in the kind of additive for anticoagulation, separation of plasma, or preservation of analyte **(Fig. 3.1)**.
- Larger tube sizes typically provide for collection of samples from 6 to 10 ml.
- Smaller collection tubes for sample sizes of 2 ml or less may be appropriate in situations where a smaller amount blood should be drawn, as in pediatric patients, or to minimize hemolysis during collection, or to avoid insufficient sample volume in the collection tube.

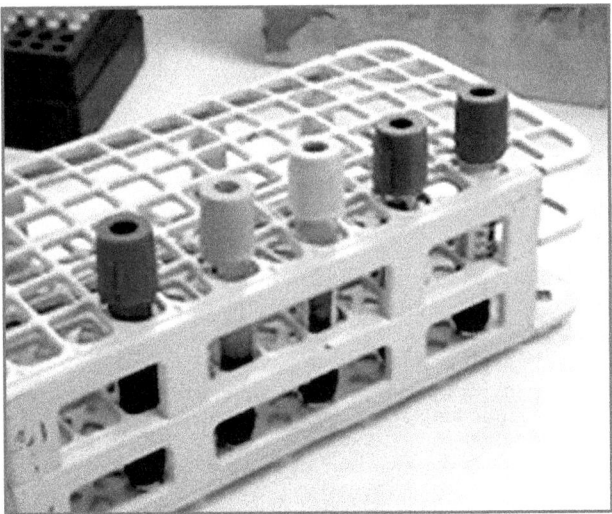

Fig. 3.1: A range of Vacutainer tubes containing blood.

BLOOD SAMPLING SYSTEM

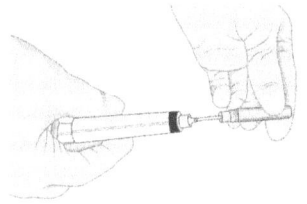
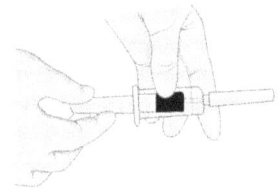

Needle and syringe system
Remove the syringe from the packaging and insert the nozzle of the syringe firmly into the exposed hub of the capped hypodermic needle

Vacuum extraction system
The barrel holds the sample collection tube in place and protects the phlebotomist from direct contact with blood. Do not push the laboratory tube onto the needle inside the barrel until the needle is in the blood vessel, or the vacuum will be lost

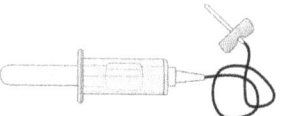
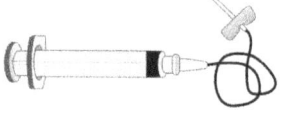

Winged butterfly system (vacuum extraction)
A vacuum system combined with a winged butterfly needle
Do not push the laboratory tube onto the needle inside the barrel until the winged needle is inside the blood vessel or the vacuum will be lost

Winged butterfly system (syringe)
A syringe combined with a winged butterfly needle

Chapter 4
SI Units and Conversion Tables

The SI units (Système International d'Unités) have replaced the old system of reporting and measurements. This is in accordance with a World Health Organization resolution which recommends the adoption of the International System of Units by the medical community throughout the world. Consequently, reports and measurements from any corner of the world can be safely understood anywhere else.

The SI system is based on metre-kilogram-second system and replaces both the foot-pound-second system and the centimetre-gram-second system. There are seven SI base units, i.e., metre, kilogram, second, mole, ampere, Kelvin and Candela. The symbols for these units and what they measure are listed in **Table 4.1**.

LITRE

The SI unit of volume is cubic metre (m^3). This is a very large unit, hence, the litre (L) although not an SI unit, has been recommended for use in the laboratory.

The litre is equal to a cubic decimetre ($1\ dm^3$). Volume measurements are made in litres or multiples and submultiples of the litre, e.g., dl (10^{-1}l), ml (10^{-3}l), µl (10^{-6}l).

Table 4.1: The symbols of units and what they measure.

SI base units			SI unit prefixes			
	Symbol	Quantity measured	Prefix	Symbol	Function	Divide by
Metre	m	length	deci	d	10^{-1}	10
Kilogram	kg	mass	centi	c	10^{-2}	100
Second	s	time	milli	m	10^{-3}	1000
Mole	mol	amount of substance	micro	µ	10^{-6}	1 000 000
Ampere	A	electric current	nano	n	10^{-9}	1 000 000 000
Kelvin	K	temperature	pico	p	10^{-12}	1 000 000 000 000
Candela	cd	luminous intensity	femto	f	10^{-15}	1 000 000 000 000 000
SI derived units						*Multiply by*
Square metre	m^2	area	deca	da	10^1	10
Cubic metre	m^3	volume	hecto	h	10^2	100
Metre per second	m/s	speed	kilo	k	10^3	1000
			mega	m	10^6	1 000 000
Named SI derived units						
Hertz	Hz	frequency	giga	G	10^9	1 000 000 000
Joule	J	energy, quantity of heat	tera	T	10^{12}	1 000 000 000 000
Newton	N	force	peta	P	10^{15}	1 000 000 000 000 000
Pascal	Pa	pressure				
Watt	W	power				
Volt	V	electric potential difference				
Degree celsius	°C	Celsius temperature				

One litre is, therefore, equivalent to 10 dl, 1000 ml or 1,000,000 µl. One dl is equivalent to 100 ml, and 1 ml to 1000 µl.

SI unit	Old unit
dl	100 ml
ml or cm^3	cc
µl	lambda
nl	—
pl	µ µl

GRAM

The kilogram (kg) is the SI unit for mass and the gram (gm) is the working unit.

Formerly, the gram (gm) was written as gramme, or gm.

Mass measurements are made in grams or in multiples and submultiples of the gram, e.g., mg (10^{-3} gm), µg (10^{-6} gm), ng (10^{-9} gm), pg (10^{-12} gm). One gm is, therefore, equivalent to 1000 mg, 1000000 µg, or 1,000,000,000 ng. One mg is equivalent to 1000 µg.

SI unit	Old unit
nm	m µ
µm	µ (micron)

MOLE (MOL)

The mole (mol) is the SI unit for amount of substance and measurements of the amounts of substances are made in moles, or in mmol (10^{-3} mol), µmol (10^{-6} mol), or nmol (10^{-9} mol).

One mol is, therefore, equivalent to 1000 mmol, 1000000 µmol, or 1000000000 nmol. One mmol/L is equivalent to 1000 µmol/L.

Earlier, the results of tests expressed in mmol/L or µmol/L were expressed in mg/100 ml or µg/100 ml. The formula used to convert mg/100 ml to mmol/L is as follows:

$$\text{mmol/L} = \frac{\text{mg/100 ml} \times 10}{\text{molecular weight of substance}}$$

where the molecular weight of a substance cannot be accurately determined (e.g., albumin), results are expressed in gm/L.

SI unit	Old unit
Mol	M
Mmol	mEq
Mmol	µM
nmol	nM

INTERNATIONAL UNIT (U)

This unit is used to express enzyme activity. An International Unit of enzyme activity is that amount of enzyme which under defined assay conditions will catalyze the conversion of 1 mmol of substrate per minute. Results are expressed in International Units per litre (U/L).

CONVERSION FACTORS BETWEEN CONVENTIONAL AND SYSTEM INTERNATIONAL UNITS (SIU)

This list is included to assist the reader to convert values between conventional units and the newer SI units that have been mandated by many journals. Only common analytes are included.

Hematology

Analyte	Conventional units	SI units	Conventional to SI units	SI to Conventional units
	Conversion factors			
WBC count (leucocytes) (B) (CSF) (SF)	µl or/cu. mm or/mm³ /cu. mm or → cu µl #/µ1	cells 10^9L 10^6/L 10^6/L #/L	0.001 1 10^6 10^6	1000 1 10^{-6} 10^{-6}
Platelet count	10^3/cu. mm	10^9/L	1	1
Reticulocytes	/cu. mm	10^9/L	0.001	1000
RBC count (erythrocytes) (B)	10^6/µl or/cu. mm	10^{12}/L	1	1
(CSF)	or/mm³/cu. mm	10^6/L	1	1
Hematocrit [packed cell volume (PCV)]	%	Volume fraction	0.01	100
Mean corpuscular volume (MCV) (volume index)	µ³ (cubic microns)	fl	1	1
Mean corpuscular hemoglobin (MCH)	pg (or µg)	pg	1	1
(color index)	pg	fmol	0.06206	16.11
Mean corpuscular hemoglobin	gm/dl	gm/L	10	0.1
concentration (MCHC)	gm/dl	mmol/L	0.6206	1.611
(Saturation index)				

Contd...

Contd...

	Conversion factors			
Analyte	Conventional units	SI units	Conventional to SI units	SI to Conventional units
Haemoglobin	gm/dl	gm/L	10	0.1
(whole blood)	gm/dl	mmol/L	0.155	6.45
(plasma)	mg/dl	µmol/L	0.155	6.45
Fetal hemoglobin	%	mol/mol	0.01	100
Haptoglobin	mg/dl	mg/L	10	0.1
Fibrinogen	mg/dl	gm/L	0.01	100

Chemistry

	Conversion factors			
Analyte	Conventional units	SI units	Conventional to SI units	SI to Conventional units
Adrenocorticotropic hormone (ACTH)	pg/ml	ng/L	1	1
	pg/ml	pmol/L	0.2202	4.541
Aldosterone				
(S)	ng/dl	nmol/L	0.0277	36.1
(U)	mEq/24 hr	mmol/d	1	1
(U)	µg/24 hr	nmol/d	2.77	0.36

Contd...

Contd...

Conversion factors

Analyte	Conventional units	SI units	Conventional to SI units	SI to Conventional units
Angiotensin	ng/dl	ng/L	10	0.1
	pg/ml	ng/L	1	1
Angiotensin-converting enzyme (ACE)	nmol/min/ml	U/L	1	1
Antidiuretic hormone (ADH) (vasopressin)	pg/ml	ng/L	1	1
Albumin				
(S)	gm/dl	gm/L	10	0.1
(CSF, AF)	mg/dl	mg/L	10	0.1
Alpha antitrypsin	mg/dl	gm/L	0.01	100
Alpha-fetoprotein (AFP)	ng/ml	µg/L	1	1
(S)	ng/dl	ng/L	10	0.1
	mg/dl	gm/L	0.01	100
	mg/dl	mg/L	10	0.1
	µg/dl	µg/L	10	0.1
Ammonia	µg/dl	µmol/L	0.714	1.4
(P)	µg/dl	µmol/L	0.5872	1.703
Anion gap	mEq/L	mmol/L	1	1
Base excess	mEq/L	mmol/L	1	1

Contd...

Contd...

Analyte	Conversion factors			
	Conventional units	SI units	Conventional to SI units	SI to Conventional units
Bicarbonate	mEq/L	mmol/L	1	1
Bilirubin	mg/dl	µmol/L	17.1	0.0584
Calcitonin	pg/ml	ng/L	1	1
Catecholamines (U)	µg/24 hr	nmol/d	5.91	0.169
Norepinephrine	µg/mg creatinine	µmol/mol creatinine	669	0.00149
	pg/ml	pmol/L	5.91	0.169
	ng/ml	nmol/L	5.91	0.169
Epinephrine	µg/24 hr	nmol/d	5.46	0.183
	µg/mg creatinine	µmol/mol creatinine	617	0.00162
	pg/ml	pmol/L	5.46	0.183
	ng/ml	nmol/L	5.46	0.183
Normetanephrine	ng/ml	nmol/L	5.46	0.183
Dopamine	µg 24 hr	nmol/d	6.53	0.153
	µg/mg creatinine	µmol/mol creatinine	783	0.00136
	pg/ml	pmol/L	6.53	0.153
	ng/ml	nmol/L	6.53	0.153
Chorionic gonadotropin (HCG), beta,	Subunit	mU/ml	IU/L	1 1
	U/24 hr	IU/d	1	1

Contd...

Contd...

<table>
<tr><th colspan="5">Conversion factors</th></tr>
<tr><th>Analyte</th><th>Conventional units</th><th>SI units</th><th>Conventional to SI units</th><th>SI to Conventional units</th></tr>
<tr><td>Calcium</td><td>mg/dl</td><td>mmol/L</td><td>0.25</td><td>4.0</td></tr>
<tr><td>(S)</td><td>mEq/L</td><td>mmol/L</td><td>0.5</td><td>2.0</td></tr>
<tr><td>(U)</td><td>mg/24 hr</td><td>mmol/d</td><td>0.025</td><td>40</td></tr>
<tr><td>Carbon dioxide total (content; CO_2 + bicarbonate)</td><td>mEq/L</td><td>mmol/L</td><td>1</td><td>1</td></tr>
<tr><td>CO_2 partial pressure, tension (PCO_2)</td><td>mmHg</td><td>kPa</td><td>0.133</td><td>7.52</td></tr>
<tr><td></td><td>mEq/L</td><td>mmol/L</td><td>1</td><td>1</td></tr>
<tr><td>Standard bicarbonate (hydrogen carbonate)</td><td>mEq/L or mg/dl</td><td>mmol/L</td><td>1</td><td>1</td></tr>
<tr><td>Chloride</td><td>ng/ml</td><td>µg/L</td><td>1</td><td>1</td></tr>
<tr><td>CEA</td><td>µg/ml</td><td>mg/L</td><td>1</td><td>1</td></tr>
<tr><td>Ceruloplasmin</td><td>mg/dl</td><td>mg/L</td><td>10</td><td>0.1</td></tr>
<tr><td>Cholesterol</td><td>mg/dl</td><td>mmol/L</td><td>0.0259</td><td>38.61</td></tr>
<tr><td>HDL-cholesterol</td><td>mg/dl</td><td>mmol/L</td><td>0.0259</td><td>38.61</td></tr>
<tr><td>LDL-cholesterol</td><td>mg/dl</td><td>mmol/L</td><td>0.0259</td><td>38.61</td></tr>
<tr><td>Copper</td><td></td><td></td><td></td><td></td></tr>
<tr><td>(S)</td><td>µg/dl</td><td>µmol/L</td><td>0.157</td><td>6.37</td></tr>
<tr><td>(U)</td><td>µg/24 hr</td><td>µmol/d</td><td>0.0157</td><td>63.69</td></tr>
<tr><td>Coproporphyrins (I and III)</td><td>µg/dl</td><td>nmol/L</td><td>15</td><td>0.067</td></tr>
</table>

Contd...

Contd...

Analyte	Conversion factors			
	Conventional units	SI units	Conventional to SI units	SI to Conventional units
(U)	µg/24 hr	nmol/d	1.5	0.67
(F)	µg/gm	nmol/gm	1.5	0.67
Porphobilinogen (PBG)				
(U)	mg/24 hr	µmol/d	4.42	0.226
Cortisol				
(S)	µg/dl	µmol/L	0.028	35.7
	ng/ml	nmol/L	2.76	0.362
17-OHKS (cortisol)	mg/24 hr	µmol/d	2.759	0.3625
(U)	µg/24 hr	nmol/d	2.759	0.3625
Creatine	mg/dl	µmol/L	76.3	0.0131
(S) Creatinine				
(S, AF)	mg/dl	µmol/L	88.4	0.0113
(U)	gm/24 hr	mmol/d	8.84	0.1131
(U)	mg/24 hr	mmol/d	0.00884	113.1
(U)	mg/kg/24 hr	µmol/kg/d	8.84	0.113
(C)	ml/min/1.73 m^2	ml/sec/m^2	0.00963	104

Contd...

Contd...

Analyte	Conversion factors			
	Conventional units	SI units	Conventional to SI units	SI to Conventional units
cAMP (cyclic adenosine monophosphate)				
(S)	µg/L	nmol/L	3.04	0.329
(B)	ng/ml	nmol/L	3.04	0.329
(U)	mg/24 hr	µmol/d	3.04	0.329
(U)	mg/gm creatinine	µmol/mol creatinine	344	0.00291
Dehydroepiandrosterone sulfate (DHEA-S)				
(S)	µg/ml	µmol/L	2.6	0.38
(AF)	ng/ml	nmol/L	2.6	0.38
17-Ketosteroids (as DHEA)				
(U)	mg/24 hr	µmol/d	3.467	0.2904
17-Ketogenic steroids (as DHEA)				
(U)	mg/24 hr	µmol/d	3.467	0.2904
17-Hydroxycorticosteroids (17-OHCS) (U)	mg/dl of creatinine	mg/mol	113.1	0.00884
11-Deoxy corticosterone (DOC)				
(S)	pg/ml	pmol/L	3.03	0.33

Contd...

Contd...

	Conversion factors			
Analyte	*Conventional units*	*SI units*	*Conventional to SI units*	*SI to Conventional units*
Glucose	mg/dl	mmol/L	0.0555	18.02
Ferritin	ng/ml	µg/L	1	1
Gastrin	pg/ml	ng/L	1	1
Growth hormone	ng/ml	µg/L	1	1
Homovanillic acid (HVA) (U)	mg/24 hr	µmol/d	5.49	0.182
	µg/24 hr	µmol/d	0.00549	182
5-Hydroxyindoleacetic acid (5-HIAA)	µg/mg of creatinine	mmol/mol of creatinine	0.621	1.61
(U)	mg/24 hr	µmol/d	5.2	0.19
Hormone receptors (T)				
Progesterone receptor assay (PRA)	fmol/mg of protein	nmol/kg of protein	1	1
Estrogen receptor assay (ERA)	fmol/mg of protein	nmol/kg of protein	1	1
Iron	µg/dl	µmol/L	0.179	5.587
Iron-binding capacity	µg/dl	µmol/L	0.179	5.587

Contd...

Contd...

	Conversion factors			
Analyte	Conventional units	SI units	Conventional to SI units	SI to Conventional units
Iron saturation	%	fraction saturation	0.01	100
Lactate	mg/dl	mmol/L	0.111	9.01
Lead				
(S)	µg/dl	µmol/L	0.0483	20.72
(S)	mg/dl	µmol/L	48.26	
(U)	µg/24 hr	µmol/d	0.00483	
Lipids (total)	mg/dl	gm/L	0.01	100
Magnesium	mEq/L	mmol/L	0.5	2
	mg/dl	mmol/L	0.411	2.433
Osmolality	mOsml/kg	same		
O_2 partial pressure (PaO_2)	mm Hg	kPa	0.133	7.5
Parathyroid hormone	pg/ml	ng/L	1	1
	µlEq/ml	mLEq/L	1	1
Phosphate (inorganic phosphorus)				
(S)	mg/dl	mmol/L	0.323	3.10
(U)	gm/24 hr	mmol/d	32.3	0.031

Contd...

Contd...

Analyte	Conventional units	SI units	Conventional to SI units	SI to Conventional units
pH	nEq/L	nmol/L	1	1
Porphobilinogen	µg/d	µmol/d	4.42	0.226
Potassium				
(S)	mEq/L	mmol/L	1	1
(U)	mEq/24 hr	mmol/L	1	1
(U)	mg/24 hr	nmol/d	0.02558	39.1
Protein, total				
(S)	gm/dl	gm/L	10	0.1
(U)	mg/24 hr	gm/d	0.001	1000
CSF	mg/dl	mg/L	10	0.1
Renin [plasma-renin activity (PRA)]	ng/ml/hr	µg/L/hr	1	1
Sodium				
(S)	mEq/L	mmol/L	1	1
(U)	mEq/24 hr	mmol/L	1	1
(U)	mg/24 hr	mmol/d	0.0435	22.99
Serotonin (S)	ng/ml	µmol/L	0.00568	176
Testosterone (total)				
(S)	ng/dl	nmol/L	0.0347	28.8

Contd...

Contd...

Analyte	Conversion factors			
	Conventional units	SI units	Conventional to SI units	SI to Conventional units
Thyroid-binding globulin (TBG)	mg/dl	mg/L	10	0.1
	µg/dl	µg/L	10	0.1
Thyroglobulin	ng/ml	µg/L	1	1
TSH (thyroid-stimulating hormone)	µU/mL	mIU/L	1	1
Thyrotropin-releasing hormone (TRH)	pg/ml	ng/L	1	1
Triiodothyronine, total (T-3)	ng/dl	nmol/L	0.0154	65.1
Reverse T-3 (rT-3)	ng/dl	nmol/L	0.0154	65.1
Thyroxine, total (T-4)	µg/dl	nmol/L	12.9	0.0775
Transferrin (TIBC)	mg/dl	gm/L	0.01	100
Triglycerides	mg/dl	mmol/L	0.0113	88.5
Urea nitrogen				
(S)	mg/dl	mmol/L	0.357	2.8
(U)	gm/24 hr	mol/d	0.0357	28
Uric acid				
(S)	mg/dl	mmol/L	0.05948	16.9
(U)	mg/24 hr	mmol/d	0.0059	169

Contd...

Contd...

Analyte	Conversion factors			
	Conventional units	SI units	Conventional to SI units	SI to Conventional units
Vanillylmandelic acid (VMA)				
(U)	mg/24 hr	µmol/d	5.05	0.198
	µg/mg of creatinine	mmol/mol of creatinine	0.571	1.75
Viscosity (S)	centipoise	same		
Vitamin B_{12} (cyanocobalamin)	pg/mL	pmol/L	0.738	1.355
Unsaturated B_{12} binding capacity				
(S)	pg/ml	pmol/L	0.738	1.355
Vitamin C (ascorbic acid)	mg/dl	µmol/L	56.78	0.176
Vitamin A	µg/dl	µmol/L	0.0349	28.65
Vitamin D (calcitriol; 1,25-dihydroxy)	pg/ml	pmol/L	2.4	0.417
Xylose (U)	mg/dl	mmol/L	0.0666	15.01
	gm/5 hr	mmol/5 hr	6.66	0.15

(µ = microns; µmol = micromoles; mmol = millimoles; nmol = nanomoles; fmol = fentamoles; mg = milligrams; gm = grams; pg = picograms; ng = nanograms; L = litre; ml = millilitre; mEq = milliequivalent; ml/sec = milliliter/second; ml/min = millilitre/minute; U = units; mU = milliunits; IU = international units; d = day; 24 hr = 24 hours; S = serum; U = urine; B = blood; C = clearance; F = feces; AF = amniotic fluid; SF = synovial fluid; T = tissue). All references are to serum unless otherwise indicated.

Enzyme

Conventional unit	IU/L equivalent
Acid phosphatase (prostatic)	
Bodansky	5.37
Shinowara-Jones-Reinhart	5.37
King-Armstrong	1.77
Bessey-Lowry-Brock	16.67
Alkaline phosphatase	
Bodansky	5.37
Shinowara-Jones-Reinhart	5.37
King-Armstrong	7.1
Bessey-Lowry-Brock	16.67
Babson	1.0
Aldolase	
Sibley-Lehninger	0.74
Amylase	
Somogyi (saccharogenic)	1.85
Somogyi	20.6
Creatine kinase (CK)	1.0
Hydroxybutyric dehydrogenase (d-HBD)	
Rosalki-Wilkinson	0.482

Contd...

Contd...

Conventional unit	IU/L equivalent
Isocitrate dehydrogenase (ICD)	
Wolfson-Williams-Ashman	0.0167
Taylor-Friedman	0.0167
Lactate dehydrogenase (LDH)	
Wroblewski	0.482
Lipase	
Cherry-Crandal	278
Malic dehydrogenase (MD)	
Wacker-Ulmer-Valee	0.482
Transaminases	
Reitman-Frankel	0.482
Karmen	0.482

Therapeutic and Toxic Drugs

	Conversion factors			
Analyte	Conventional units	SI units	Conventional to SI units	SI to conventional units
Acetaminophen	µg/ml	µmol/L	6.62	0.151
Amikacin	µg/ml	µmol/L	1.71	0.585

Contd...

Contd...

	Conversion factors			
Analyte	Conventional units	SI units	Conventional to SI units	SI to conventional units
Amitriptyline	ng/ml	nmol/L	3.61	0.277
Amobarbital	µg/ml	µmol/L	4.42	0.226
Amphetamine	ng/ml	nmol/L	7.4	0.135
	µg/ml	µmol/L	7.4	0.135
Bromide	µg/ml	mmol/L	0.0125	79.9
Caffeine	µg/ml	µmol/L	5.15	0.194
Carbamazepine (Tegretol)	µg/ml	µmol/L	4.23	0.236
Carbenicillin	µg/ml	µmol/L	2.64	0.378
Chloral hydrate	µg/ml	µmol/L	6.69	0.149
Chloramphenicol	µg/ml	µmol/L	3.09	0.323
Chlordiazepoxide (Librium)	ng/ml	µmol/L	0.00334	300
Chlorpromazine (Thorazine)	ng/ml	nmol/L	3.14	0.319
Chlorpropamide (Diabinese)	µg/ml	µmol/L	3.61	0.227
Cimetidine (Tagamet)	µg/ml	µmol/L	3.96	0.252

Contd...

Contd...

<table>
<tr><th colspan="5">Conversion factors</th></tr>
<tr><th>Analyte</th><th>Conventional units</th><th>SI units</th><th>Conventional to SI units</th><th>SI to conventional units</th></tr>
<tr><td>Clonazepam (Clonopin)</td><td>ng/ml</td><td>nmol/L</td><td>3.17</td><td>0.316</td></tr>
<tr><td>Clonidine (Catapres)</td><td>ng/ml</td><td>nmol/L</td><td>4.35</td><td>0.230</td></tr>
<tr><td>Cocaine</td><td>ng/ml</td><td>nmol/L</td><td>3.3</td><td>0.303</td></tr>
<tr><td>Codeine</td><td>ng/ml</td><td>nmol/L</td><td>3.34</td><td>0.299</td></tr>
<tr><td>Demerol (Meperidine)</td><td>ng/ml</td><td>nmol/L</td><td>4.04</td><td>0.247</td></tr>
<tr><td>Desipramine (Norpramin)</td><td>ng/ml</td><td>nmol/L</td><td>3.75</td><td>0.267</td></tr>
<tr><td>Diazepam (Valium)</td><td>ng/ml</td><td>µmol/L</td><td>0.0035</td><td>285</td></tr>
<tr><td>Digitoxin</td><td>ng/ml</td><td>nmol/L</td><td>1.31</td><td>0.765</td></tr>
<tr><td>Digoxin</td><td>ng/ml</td><td>nmol/L</td><td>1.28</td><td>0.781</td></tr>
<tr><td>Dilaudid</td><td>ng/ml</td><td>nmol/L</td><td>4.85</td><td>0.206</td></tr>
<tr><td>Disulfiram</td><td>µg/ml</td><td>µmol/L</td><td>12.12</td><td>0.0761</td></tr>
<tr><td>Doxepin (Sinequan)</td><td>ng/ml</td><td>nmol/L</td><td>3.58</td><td>0.279</td></tr>
<tr><td>Ethanol</td><td>mg/dl</td><td>mmol/L</td><td>0.217</td><td>4.61</td></tr>
<tr><td>Ethchlorvynol (Placidyl)</td><td>µg/ml</td><td>µmol/L</td><td>6.92</td><td>0.145</td></tr>
<tr><td>Ethosuximide (Zarontin)</td><td>µg/ml</td><td>µmol/L</td><td>7.08</td><td>0.141</td></tr>
</table>

Contd...

Contd...

	Conversion factors			
Analyte	Conventional units	SI units	Conventional to SI units	SI to conventional units
Gentamicin	μg/ml	μmol/L	2.09	0.478
Glutethimide (Doriden)	μg/ml	μmol/L	4.60	0.217
Haloperidol (Haldol)	ng/ml	nmol/L	2.66	0.376
Ibuprofen	μg/ml	μmol/L	4.85	0.206
Imipramine (Tofranil)	ng/ml	nmol/L	3.57	0 28
Isoniazid	μg/ml	μmol/L	7.29	0.137
Kanamycin (Kantrex)	μg/ml	μmol/L	2.06	0.485
Lidocaine (Xylocaine)	μg/ml	μmol/L	4.27	0.234
Lithium	mEq/L	mmol/L	1	1
Lorazepam	ng/ml	nmol/L	3.11	0.321
LSD (lysergic acid diethylamide)	μg/ml	μmol/L	3.09	0.323
Meprobamate	mg/L	μmol/L	4.58	0.218
Methadone	ng/ml	μmol/L	0.00323	309
Methaqualone (Quaalude)	μg/ml	μmol/L	4.0	0.250
Methotrexate	ng/ml	nmol/L	2.2	0.454

Contd...

Contd...

	Conversion factors			
Analyte	Conventional units	SI units	Conventional to SI units	SI to conventional units
Methsuximide	µg/ml	µmol/L	5.29	0.189
Methyldopa (Aldomet)	µg/ml	µmol/L	4.73	0.211
Morphine	ng/ml	nmol/L	3.5	0.285
	ng/ml	µmol/L	0.0035	285
Nortriptyline	ng/ml	nmol/L	3.8	0.263
Oxazepam	µg/ml	µmol/L	3.49	0.287
Paraldehyde	µg/ml	µmol/L	7.57	0.132
Pentobarbital (Nembutal)	µg/ml	µmol/L	4.42	0.179
Percodan	ng/ml	nmol/L	3.17	0.315
Phenacetin	µg/ml	µmol/L	5.58	0.179
Phenobarbital (Luminal)	µg/ml	µmol/L	4.31	0.232
Phenylbutazone (Butazolidin)	µg/ml	µmol/L	3.08	0.324
Phenytoin (Dilantin)	µg/ml	µmol/L	3.96	0.253
Primidone	µg/ml	µmol/L	4.58	0.218
Procainamide (Pronestyl), procaine	µg/ml	µmol/L	4.23	0.236

Contd...

Contd...

	Conversion factors			
Analyte	Conventional units	SI units	Conventional to SI units	SI to conventional units
Propoxyphene (Darvon)	µg/ml	µmol/L	3.07	0.326
Propranolol	ng/ml	nmol/L	3.86	0.259
Quinidine	µg/ml	µmol/L	3.08	0.324
Quinine	µg/ml	µmol/L	3.08	0.324
Salicylic acid	µg/ml	µmol/L	7.24	0.138
Secobarbital (Seconal)	µg/ml	µmol/L	4.2	0.238
Theophylline (Aminophylline)	µg/ml	µmol/L	5.55	0.180
Tobramycin	µg/ml	µmol/L	2.14	0.467
Valproic acid	µg/ml	µmol/L	6.93	0.144
Vancomycin	µg/ml	mg/L	1	1
Warfarin (Coumadin)	µg/ml	µmol/L	3.24	0.308

Chapter 5

Body Excreta Analysis

URINE ANALYSIS

COMPOSITION OF URINE

Urine composition is affected mainly by three factors:
1. Nutritional status
2. State of metabolic processes
3. Ability of the kidney to selectively handle the material presented to it.

Physicochemical Characteristics of Urine

Dry weight	55–70 gm/24 hr
Osmolality	38–1400 mOsm/kg water
	(Average = 500–800 mOsm/kg water)
pH	4.6–8.0 (mean = 6.1)

Specific gravity

Neonates	1.012
Infants	1.002–1.006
Adults	1.003–1.030

Volume:	*Per day*
Neonates	30–60 ml
10–60 days	250–450 ml
60–365 days	400–500 ml
Children	
1–3 years	500–600 ml
3–5 years	600–700 ml
5–8 years	650–1000 ml
8–14 years	800–1400 ml
Adults	600–2500 ml (Avg: 1200 ml)

Inorganic Constituents per 24 Hours

Iron	0.06–0.1 mg
Chlorides	6 (4–10) gm on usual diet
Sodium	4 gm on usual diet
Phosphate	0.8–1.3 gm on usual diet
Sulphur	2 gm
Calcium	< 150 mg.

Organic Constituents per 24 Hours

Nitrogenous—total	25–35 gm
Urea	15–30 gm
Creatinine	1.4 (1–1.8) gm
Ammonia	0.7 (0.3–1) gm
Uric acid	0.45 (0.3–0.6) gm
Protein (albumin)	0–0.1 gm

Creatine, in children: 10–50 mg (Excreted in urine in adults in hepatic or muscle disorders or thyrotoxicosis).

Glucose fasting range: 2–20 mg% (Diabetic may lose up to 100 gm/day)
Amylase (diastase): 40–260 units/hour.

Cells and Casts

	As per Addis count	
	Range	Mean
RBC	Up to 1 million /day (more in females)	130,000/day
Casts		
Hyaline and occasionally granular	Up to 5,000/day	2,000/day
Leucocytes	Up to 5 million /hour (more in females)	108,000/hr, females; 28,000/hr, males
Epithelial cells	Up to 2.5 lakh/hour (more in males)	68,000/hr, females; 78,000/ hr, males
Squamous cells epithelial	Variable	

Collection of Urine

The urine sample should be collected in a clean, dry container and should be examined fresh. For cultures sterile containers should be used. With time, RBC, and leucocytes tend to be destroyed due to hypotonicity of the urine. Casts too tend to get decomposed. Bacterial contamination of stale urine is frequent and causes alkalinization of the urine due to conversion of urea to ammonia and loss of glucose. This rise in pH accelerates loss of leucocytes and epithelial cells. For ordinary qualitative tests a random sample is enough. For diabetes mellitus, a 2 hours postprandial sample is desirable; for nephritis, a morning specimen is best as it has higher specific gravity and lower pH desirable for preservation of formed elements.

Repeated samples are necessary sometimes, as for orthostatic proteinuria.

Whenever needed, a 24-hour urine should be collected in a large container. Have patient void and discard urine at any particular time, save all urine for the next 24-hours, and then void at the same hour to finish the collection.

Preservation of Specimen

Urinary decomposition occurs quickly in warm temperatures. Hence, fresh specimens should be examined, if not, then it should be refrigerated. As far as possible, the need for preservation should not arise. However, the following preservatives can be used:
- *Toluol:* Best for preservation of chemical constituents. Add 2 mL toluol/100 mL urine.
- *Thymol:* A small floating lump of thymol can preserve the urine for several days in a bottle. Thymol may, however, cause a false-positive reaction for protein.
- *Formalin:* 1 drop/30 mL urine is good for preserving formed elements. It can precipitate proteins and can reduce Benedict's solution.
- *Boric acid:* 0.3 g/120 mL of urine. However, yeasts can still grow and uric acid crystals get precipitated.

GROSS EXAMINATION OF URINE

Color and Appearance

Normal urine is clear and pale yellow (straw) in color.
- *Colorless:* Dilution; diabetes mellitus/insipidus, nervousness, diuretic or alcohol intake.

- *Milky:* Purulent genitourinary tract disease; chyluria.
- *Orange:* Urobilinogenuria, fever, excessive sweating, concentrated urine.
- *Red:* Beetroot ingestion, hematuria, hemoglobinuria, phenolphthalein, pyridium, sulfonal.
- *Greenish:* Jaundice, phenol poisoning.
- *Dirty blue or green:* Putrefying urine, in typhus or cholera, methylene blue.
- *Dark brown, brown red, or yellow:* Very concentrated urine. Acute febrile diseases. Bilirubinuria.
- *Brown-yellow or brown-red (if acidic) or bright red (if alkaline):* Due to rhubarb, cascara, aloes.
- *Brown, brown black or black:* Hemorrhage in urinary tract if urine is acidic (Acid-hematin); hemoglobinuria; porphyria, methemoglobinuria; myoglobinuria, melanin, phenol poisoning, homogentisic acid (alkaptonuria). In porphyria, urine turns dark brown on exposure to sunlight or boiling.

Interfering Factors

- Normally, urine darkens on standing. This occurs because of oxidation of urobilinogen to urobilin. Decomposition of urine commences in half an hour.
- Some foods cause change in urine color
  - Beets turn the urine red
  - Rhubarb changes color of urine to brown
- Many drugs are also responsible for urinary color change
  - Cascara and senna laxatives in acidic urine will turn the urine reddish-brown, in alkaline urine they will turn the urine red
  - Phenazopyridine (pyridium), amidopyrine turn urine orange in color

- Pyridium, ethoxazene turn urine to orange/orange red
- Orange to purple red may occur due to chlorzoxazone
- Salicylazosulfapyridine, anisindone, or phenindione turn urine color to orange-yellow in alkaline urine
- Sulphonamides and nitrofurantoins produce rust-yellow to brownish color
- Dilantin (dephenydantoin) dioctyl calcium sulphosuccinate, phenolphthalein and phenothiazine turn urine color to pink to red or red-brown
- Phenolphthalein may also produce magenta color
- Amidopyrine, pyridium, aniline dyes, BSP, PSP in alkaline urine or phenolphthalein and pyridium in acid urine or deferoxamine can produce red urine.
- Phenolphthalein in alkaline urine produces purple red color
- Phenylhydrazine and phenolic drugs produce dark brown urine
- Cascara may produce brown-black urine
- Riboflavin or pyridium in alkaline urine produce bright yellow color
- Methylene blue and amitriptyline produce blue or green colored urine
- Levodopa causes urine to darken on standing
- Iron salt consumption produces dark colored urine
- Phenothiazine tranquilizers cause pink to brown color
- Triameterene causes pale blue colored urine.

Reaction

Average range: 4.6–8, Average pH = 6.0

Litmus paper or other pH indicator papers broad range (pH 1–12) or narrow range pH papers can be used. Another simple method is to add 2 drops of 0.4% alcoholic solution of methyl red to 5 mL of urine. Note the color change—if red = acidic; orange = neutral; yellow = alkaline. Digital electronic pH meters for better accuracy can be used—here, the electrode is dipped in urine and pH is read off directly from the digital display.

Amongst urinary tract infections, *Escherichia coli* produces acidic urine, while *Proteus* (urea splitting) produces alkaline urine. Meat protein diet causes urinary acidification, while consumption of citrus fruits makes the urine alkaline.

Urine pH

Finding and condition	Causes and comments
Acidic urine	
Ketosis	Diabetes, starvation, febrile illness in children
Systemic acidosis	Except with impaired renal tubular function, respiratory or metabolic acidosis provokes intense urine acidity and decreased NH^+ excretion.
Acidification	Used in treating urinary tract infections, and to prevent precipitation of calcium carbonate or phosphates or magnesium ammonium phosphate.
Alkaline urine	
Postprandial Alkaline tide Vegetarianism	Normal finding in specimens voided shortly after meals. Meats produce fixed acid residue, vegetarian diet does not.
Systemic	As may occur in severe vomiting, hyperventilation, excess alkali ingestion.

Contd...

Contd...

Finding and condition	Causes and comments
Urinary tract infection	Proteus or Pseudomonas infections, they split urea to HCO_3^- and ammonia.
Alkalinization	Used to prevent crystallization of uric acid, oxalate, cystine, sulphonamides, streptomycin.
Stale specimen	Bacterial overgrowth. If true infection exists, the sediment should show pus cells.
Renal tubular	Impaired tubular acidification causes inappropriately high urine pH with systemic acidosis and low serum HCO_3^-

Interfering Factors

- On standing, urinary pH becomes alkaline because CO_2 will diffuse into the air
- Alkaline urine specimens tend to cause hemolysis of red cells and disappearance of casts
- High protein diets will cause excessively acidic urine
- Ammonium chloride and mandelic acid may produce acidic urines
- Alkaline urine after meals is a normal response to the secretions of HCl in gastric juices
- Sodium bicarbonate, potassium citrate, and acetazolamide may produce alkaline urines.

Be Careful

- Only a freshly voided sample is suitable for measuring pH. Refrigerate the sample if any delay is expected

- Alkaline urine occurs from vegetarian diets, citrus fruits, milk and other dairy products
- Highly concentrated urine such as that formed in hot, dry environments is strongly acidic and may be irritating
- While sleeping, decreased pulmonary ventilation causes respiratory acidosis and urine becomes highly acidic
- Chlorothiazide diuretic will cause acidic urine to be excreted
- Bacterial contamination and overgrowth will result in alkaline urine. Bacteria in urine will convert to ammonia.

Odor

Important in fresh specimens only and is aromatic because of volatile fatty acids. Bacterial action causes ammoniacal odor, while ketosis leads to a fruity odor in urine.

Specific Gravity

Specific gravity depends upon the concentration of various solutes in the urine.

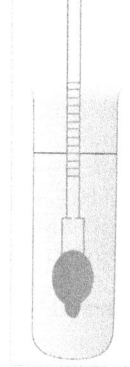

- *Urinometre:* Urine should be foamless. Transfer urine (about 70-80 mL) into the urinometre container and let the urinometre float freely without touching the sides or the bottom of the container (**Fig. 5.1**). Read graduations at the lowest level of urinary meniscus. If the urine amount is less, dilute the urine to raise the volume till 70-80 mL, take the reading and multiply the last two digits by the dilution factor.
- *Refractometre:* Only small amount of urine is needed. It measures the concentration of

Fig. 5.1: Urinometre.

solutes (related to refractive index). In Goldberg refractometre the specific gravity of urine can be read directly from the calibration.
- Can be tested with *Dipstick* also.
- *Osmometry:* Gives the most accurate assessment.

Correction factor for temperature: While using urinometer, add or subtract 0.001 for each 3°C above or below the standardization temperature of the instrument.

Urines of low specific gravity are called hyposthenuric (< 1.007) while urines of fixed specific gravity of about 1.010 are known as isothenuric.

High specific gravity
- Excessive sweating
- Glycosuria
- Acute nephritis
- Albuminuria
- All causes of oliguria.

Low specific gravity (less than 1.010)
- Excessive water intake
- Chronic nephritis
- Diabetes insipidus
- All causes of polyuria except diabetes mellitus.

Low and fixed specific gravity (1.010 to 1.012)
- Chronic nephritis (end-stage kidney) when concentration power of renal tubules is low
- ADH deficiency
- Arteriosclerotic kidney.

Interfering Factors

- Specific gravity is maximum in the first morning sample
- Specific gravity is increased whenever there is an excessive loss of water. It occurs in:
  - Sweating
  - Fever
  - Vomiting
  - Diarrhea
- Drugs leading to false-positive:
  - Dextran
  - Radiopaque contrast media used in X-rays of the urinary tract.
- Temperature of urine specimens affects specific gravity when specific gravity is measured in urine removed from the refrigerator. Specific gravity will be falsely higher.
- Reagent strip testing of urine containing glycosuria greater than 1% may cause a low specific gravity. Highly buffered alkaline urine may also cause a low reading.
- Elevated reading may occur in presence of moderate (100–750 mg/dl) amounts of proteinuria.

Urinary Volume

The average 24 hour urinary output in an adult is around 1200 to 1500 mL and the night urine should not be more than 400 mL.

A volume more than 2000 mL is termed polyuria. Oliguria implies excretion of urine less than 500 mL and anuria is complete cessation. Nocturia is excretion by an adult of urine more than 500 mL with a specific gravity of less than 1.018 at night (characteristic of chronic glomerulonephritis).

Polyuria

- Neurotic polydipsia
- Diabetes mellitus/insipidus
- Diuretics
- Intravenous saline/glucose
- Chronic renal failure
- Addison's disease, decrease of adrenocortical hormones.

Oliguria

- Dehydration:
    - Vomiting
    - Diarrhea
    - Excessive sweating
- Renal ischemia
- Acute renal tubular necrosis
- Acute glomerulonephritis
- Obstruction to urinary outflow.

Turbidity

Normally—fresh urine is clear.

The appearance of cloudy urine provides a warning of possible abnormalities such as the presence of pus, RBCs or bacteria. Sometimes, however, excretion of cloudy urine may not be abnormal since the change in urine pH may cause precipitation within the bladder of normal urinary constituents. Alkaline urine may appear cloudy because of presence of phosphates, and urine may appear cloudy because of urates.

- Pathologic urines are often turbid or cloudy, but so are many normal urines. Cloudy urine may appear from precipitation of crystals due to rapid cooling of the urine.

- Occasionally, urine turbidity may result from urinary tract infections.
- Abnormal urines may be cloudy on account of presence of RBCs, pus cells or bacteria.

Interfering Factors

- After ingestion of food, urates or phosphates may produce cloudiness in normal urine.
- Vaginal contamination in female patients is often a cause of turbidity
- Greasy cloudiness may be caused by lipiduria
- Many normal urines will develop haziness or turbidity after being refrigerated or on standing at room temperature.

Rapid Diagnostics

Rapidity of diagnosis is of utmost importance in today's context.

Many manufacturers now provide rapid strip tests (qualitative and semiquantitative). Important amongst them are as follows.

Strip Tests from Boehringer-Knoll Limited

Product	Determines
A. Combur 9 test	• Leucocytes, nitrite, pH, protein, glucose, ketone bodies, urobilinogen, bilirubin, blood
B. Combur 8 test	• All of A except leucocytes
C. Combur 7 test	• All of B except nitrite
D. Combur 6 test	• All of C except bilirubin
E. Combur 4 test	• Protein, glucose urobilinogen, blood
F. Ecur test	• Protein, glucose, blood
G. Combur test	• Glucose, protein, pH

Various other combinations or single test strips are also available, e.g., pertaining only to liver/kidney disorders.

Strip Tests from Bayer India Limited

Now with improved pad order and efficacy.

Product	Determines
A. Diastix	◆ Glucose
B. Hemastix	◆ Blood
C. Ictotest (tablets)	◆ Bilirubin
D. Keto-diastix	◆ Glucose and ketones pH
E. Multistix	◆ Protein, glucose, ketones, bilirubin, blood, urobilinogen
F. Uristix	◆ Glucose and protein
G. Combistix SG	◆ Glucose, protein, pH and specific gravity
H. Multistix SG	◆ All of E + Specific gravity
I. Neostix 3	◆ Blood, glucose and protein

MULTIPLE® REAGENT STRIPS FOR URINALYSIS

Tests for Glucose, Bilirubin, Ketone (Acetoacetic Acid), Specific Gravity, Blood, pH, Protein and Urobilinogen in Urine. Refer to the carton and bottle label for specific reagent areas on the product you are using.

Summary and Explanation/Intended Use

Bayer Reagent strips for urinalysis are firm plastic strips to which are affixed several separate reagent areas. Depending on the product being used, Bayer Reagent strips provide tests for glucose, bilirubin, ketone (acetoacetic acid). specific gravity, blood, pH, protein, and urobilinogen in urine. *Please refer to the carton and bottle label for specific reagent areas on the product you are using.* Test results may provide information regarding the status of carbohydrate metabolism, kidney and liver function, and acid-base balance.

The reagent test areas on Bayer Reagent strips are ready to use upon removal from the bottle and the entire reagent strip is disposable. The strips may be read visually, requiring no additional laboratory equipment for testing. Certain configurations of strips may also be read instrumentally, using the CLINITEK® family of urine chemistry analyzers and the appropriate program module or program card.

The directions must be followed exactly. Accurate timing is essential to provide optimal results. The reagent strips must be kept in the bottle with the cap tightly closed to maintain reagent reactivity. To obtain optimal results, it is necessary to use fresh, well-mixed, uncentrifuged urine.

Chemical Principles of the Procedure

Glucose

This test is based on a double sequential enzyme reaction. One enzyme, glucose oxidase, catalyzes the formation of gluconic acid and hydrogen peroxide from the oxidation of glucose. A second enzyme, peroxidase, catalyzes the reaction of hydrogen peroxide with a potassium iodide chromogen to oxidize the chromogen to colors ranging from green to brown.

Bilirubin

This test is based on the coupling of bilirubin with diazotized dichloroaniline in a strongly acid medium. The color ranges through various shades of tan.

Ketone

This test is based on the development of colors ranging from buff-pink, for a negative reading, to purple when acetoacetic acid reacts with nitroprusside.

Specific Gravity

This test is based on the apparent pKa change of certain pretreated polyelectrolytes in relation to ionic concentration. In the presence of an indicator, colors range from deep blue-green in urine of low ionic concentration through green and yellow-green in urines of increasing ionic concentration.

Blood

This test is based on the peroxidase-like activity of hemoglobin, which catalyzes the reaction of disopropylbenzene dihydroperoxide and 3.3', 5,5'-tetramenthylbenzidine. The resulting color ranges from orange through green; very high levels of blood may cause the color development to continue to blue.

pH

The test is based on the double indicator principle that gives a broad range of color covering the entire urinary pH range. Colors range from orange through yellow and green to blue.

Protein

This test is based on the **protein error indicators** principle. At a constant pH, the development of any green color is due to the presence of protein. Colors range from yellow for "Negative" through yellow-green and green to green-blue for "Positive" reactions.

Urobilinogen

This test is based on a modified Ehrlich reaction, in which p-diethylaminobenzaldehyde in conjunction with a color enhancer reacts with urobilinogen in a strongly acid medium to produce a pink-red color.

Reagents

Based on dry weight at time of impregnation.

Glucose

2.2% w/w glucose oxidase (microbial, 1.3 IU); 1.0% w/w peroxidase (horseradish, 3300 IU); 8.1% w/w potassium iodide; 69.8% w/w buffer; 18.9% w/w nonreactive ingredients.

Bilirubin

0.4% w/w 2, 4–dichloroaniline diazonium salt; 37.3% w/w buffer; 62.3% w/w nonreactive ingredients.

Ketone

7.1% w/w sodium nitroprusside; 92.9% w/w buffer.

Specific Gravity

2.8% w/w bromothymol blue; 68.8% w/w poly (methyl vinyl ether/maleic anhydride); 28.4% w/w sodium hydroxide.

Blood

6.8% w/w diisopropylbenzene dihydroperoxide; 4.0% w/w 3.3', 5,5'-tetramethylbenzidine; 48.0% w/w buffer; 41.2% w/w nonreactive ingredients.

pH

1.2% w/w methyl red; 2.8% w/w bromothymol blue; 97.0% w/w nonreactive ingredients.

Protein

1.3% w/w tetrabromophenol blue; 97.3% w/w buffer; 2.4% w/w nonreactive ingredients.

Urobilinogen

0.2% w/w ρ-diethylaminobenzaldehyde; 99.8% w/w nonreactive ingredients.

Warning and Precautions

Bayer reagent strips are for in vitro diagnostic use.

Storage

Storage below 30°C in a cool, dry place. Do not refrigerate. Keep out of direct sunlight. Do not use after expiration date.

Recommended Procedures for Handling Bayer Reagent Strips

All unused strips must remain in the original bottle. Transfer to any other container may cause reagent strips to deteriorate and become unreactive. Do not remove desiccant(s) from bottle. **Do not remove strip from the bottle until immediately before it is to be used for testing. Replace cap immediately and tightly after removing reagent strip. Do not touch test areas of the reagent strip.** Work areas and specimen containers should be free of detergents and other contaminating substances.

Dip test areas in urine completely, but briefly, to avoid dissolving out the reagent. If using strips visually, read test results carefully at the time specified, in a good light (such as fluorescent) and with the test area held near the appropriate color chart on the bottle label. Do not read the strips in direct sunlight. If the strips are used instrumentally, carefully follow the directions given in the appropriate instrument operating manual.

Important

Protection against ambient moisture, light and heat is essential to guard against altered reagent reactivity. Discoloration or darkening of reagent areas may indicate deterioration. If this is evident, or if test results are questionable or inconsistent with expected findings, the following steps are recommended:

- Confirm that the product is within the expiration date shown on the label.
- Check performance against known negative and positive control materials (e.g., CHEK- STIX** Control Strips);
- Retest with fresh product. If proper results are not obtained, consult your local product representative for advice on testing technique and results.

Specimen Collection and Preparation

Collect urine in a clean container and test it as soon as possible. Do not centrifuge. The use of urine preservatives is not recommended. If testing cannot be done within an hour after voiding, refrigerate the specimen immediately and let it return to room temperature before testing.

It is especially important to use fresh urine to obtain optimal results with the tests for bilirubin and urobilinogen, as these compounds are very unstable when exposed to room temperature and light.

Prolonged exposure of urine to room temperature may result in microbial proliferation with resultant changes in pH. A shift to alkaline pH may cause false positive results with the protein test area. Urine containing glucose may decrease in pH as organisms metabolize the glucose. Bacterial growth from contaminating organisms may cause false positive blood reactions from the peroxidases produced.

Contamination of the urine specimen with skin cleansers containing chlorhexidine may affect protein (and to a lesser extent specific gravity and bilirubin) test results. The user should determine whether the use of such skin cleansers is warranted.

Procedure

Must be followed exactly to achieve reliable test results.

- Collect FRESH urine specimen in a clean, dry container. Mix well immediately before testing.
- Remove one strip from bottle and replace cap. Completely immerse reagent areas of the strip in fresh urine and remove immediately to avoid dissolving out reagents.
- While removing, run the edge of the entire length of the strip against the rim of the urine container to remove excess urine. Hold the strip in a horizontal position to prevent possible mixing of chemicals from adjacent reagent areas and/or contaminating the hands with urine.
  - If reading visually, compare reagent areas to corresponding Color Chart on the bottle label at the times specified. *Hold strip close to color blocks and match carefully.* Avoid lying

the strip directly on the Color Chart, as this will result in the urine soiling the chart.
- If reading instrumentally, carefully follow the directions given in the appropriate instrument operating manual.

Proper read time is critical for optimal results. If using strips visually, read the glucose and bilirubin tests at 30 seconds after dipping. Read the ketone test at 40 seconds; the specific gravity test at 45 seconds; pH, protein, urobilinogen and blood at 60 seconds. The pH and protein areas may also be read immediately or at any time up to 2 minutes after dipping.

After dipping the strip, check the pH area. If the color on the pad is not uniform, read the reagent area immediately, comparing the darkest color to the appropriate Color Chart. All reagent areas may be read between 1 and 2 minutes for identifying negative specimens and for determination of the pH and SG. Color changes that occur after 2 minutes are of no diagnostic value. If using strips instrumentally, the instrument will automatically read each reagent area at a specified time.

Results

Results with Bayer Reagent Strips are obtained in clinically meaningful units directly from the Color Chart comparison when using strips visually. With instrumental use, the reagent pads are "read" by the instrument and the results are displayed or printed. The color blocks and instrumental display values represent nominal values; actual values will vary around the nominal values.

Limitations of Procedures

As with all laboratory tests, definitive diagnostic or therapeutic decisions should not be based on any single result or method.

Substances that cause abnormal urine color, such as drugs containing Azo dyes (e.g., Pyridium®, Azo Gantrisin®, Azo Gantanol®), nitrofurantoin (Macrodantin®, Furadantin®), and riboflavin, may affect the readability of the reagent areas on urinalysis reagent strips. The color development on the reagent pad may be masked, or a color reaction may be produced on the pad that could be interpreted visually and/or instrumentally as a false positive.

Glucose

Ascorbic acid concentrations of 50 mg/dl or greater may cause false negatives for specimens containing small amounts of glucose (75–125 mg/dL). Ketone bodies reduce the sensitivity of the test; moderately high ketone levels (40 mg/dl) may cause false negatives for specimens containing small amounts of glucose (75–125 mg/dl) but the combination of such ketone levels and low glucose levels is metabolically improbable in screening. The reactivity of the glucose test decreases as the SG of the urine increases. Reactivity may also vary with temperature.

Bilirubin

Indican (Indoxyl sulfate) can produce a yellow-orange to red color response that may interfere with the interpretation of a negative or a positive bilirubin reading. Metabolites of Lodine® (etodolac) may cause false positive or atypical results; ascorbic acid concentrations of 25 mg/dl or greater may cause false negatives. Since very small amounts of bilirubin may be found in the earliest phases of liver disease, the user must consider whether the sensitivity of Bayer Reagent Strips to bilirubin is sufficient for the intended use.

Ketone

False positive results (Trace or less) may occur with highly pigmented urine specimens or those containing large amounts of levodopa metabolites. Compounds such as mesna (2-mercapto-ethane sulfonic acid) that contain sulfhydryl groups may cause false positive results or an atypical color reaction.

Specific Gravity

The chemical nature of the Bayer SG test may cause slightly different results from those obtained with other specific gravity methods when elevated amounts of certain urine consti- tuents are present. Highly buffered alkaline urines may cause low readings relative to other methods. Elevated specific gravity readings may be obtained in the presence of moderate quantities (100–750 mg/dl) of protein.

Blood

Elevated specific gravity may reduce the reactivity of the blood test. Clapoten® (captopril) may also cause decreased reactivity. Certain oxidizing contaminants, such as hypochlorite, may produce false positive results. Microbial peroxidase associated with urinary tract infection may cause a false positive reaction. Levels of ascorbic acid normally found in urine do not interfere with this test.

pH

If proper procedure is not followed and excess urine remains on the strip, a phenomenon known as "runover" may occur, in which the acid buffer from the protein reagent will run onto the pH area, causing a false lowering of the pH result.

Protein

False positive results may be obtained with highly buffered or alkaline urines. Contamination of the urine specimen with quaternary ammonium compounds (e.g., from some antiseptics and detergents) or with skin cleansers containing chlorhexidine may also produce false positive results.

Urobilinogen

The reagent area may react with interfering substances known to react with Ehrlich's reagent, such as p-aminosalicylic acid and sulfonamides. Atypical color reactions may be obtained in the presence of high concentrations of ρ-aminobenzoic acid. False negative results may be obtained if formalin is present. Strip reactivity increases with temperature; the optimum temperature is 22–26°C. The test is not a reliable method for the detection of porphobilinogen. The absence of urobilinogen cannot be determined with this test.

Expected Values

Expected values for the typical "normal" healthy population and the abnormal population are listed below for each reagent. Exact agreement between visual results and instrumental results might not be found because of the inherent differences between the perception of the human eye and the optical systems of the instruments.

Glucose

Small amounts of glucose are normally excreted by the kidney. These amounts are usually below the sensitivity of this test but on occasion may produce a color between the negative and the

100 mg/dl color blocks, and that is interpreted by the instrument as a positive result. Results at the first positive level may be significantly abnormal if found consistently.

Bilirubin

Normally no bilirubin is detectable in urine by even the most sensitive methods. Even trace amounts of bilirubin are sufficiently abnormal to require further investigation. Atypical colors (colors that are unlike the negative or positive color blocks shown on the Color Chart) may indicate that bilirubin-derived bile pigments are present in the urine sample and may be masking the bilirubin reaction. These colors may indicate bile pigment abnormalities and the urine specimen should be tested further.

Ketone

Normal urine specimens ordinarily yield negative results with this reagent. Detectable levels of ketone may occur in urine during physiological stress conditions such as fasting, pregnancy and frequent strenuous exercise. In ketoacidosis, starvation or with other abnormalities of carbohydrate or lipid metabolism, ketones may appear in urine in large amounts before serum ketone concentrations are elevated.

Specific Gravity

Random urines may vary in specific gravity from 1.001–1.035. Twenty-four-hour urines from normal adults with normal diets and normal fluid intake will have a specific gravity of 1.016–1.022.

Blood

The significance of the Trace reaction may vary among patients, and clinical judgment is required for assessment in an individual case. Development of green spots (intact erythrocytes) or green color (free hemoglobin/myoglobin) on the reagent area within 60 seconds indicates the need for further investigation. Blood is often, but not always, found in the urine of menstruating females. This test is highly sensitive to hemoglobin and thus complements the microscopic examination.

pH

Both the normal and abnormal urinary pH range is from 5 to 9.

Protein

Normally no protein is detectable in urine, although a minute amount is excreted by the normal kidney. A color matching any block greater than Trace indicates significant proteinuria. For urine of high specific gravity, the test area may most closely match the Trace color block even though only normal concentrations of protein are present. Clinical judgment is needed to evaluate the significance of Trace results.

Urobilinogen

The normal urobilinogen range obtained with this test is 0.2 to 1.0 mg/dl. A result of 2.0 mg/dl represents the transition from normal to abnormal, and the patient and/or urine specimen should be evaluated further.

The following table lists the generally detectable levels of analytes in contrived urine; however, because of the inherent variability of clinical urines, lesser concentrations may be detected under certain conditions.

Reagent area	Sensitivity
• Glucose	• 75–125 mg/dl glucose
• Bilirubin	• 0.4–0.8 mg/dl bilirubin
• Ketone	• 5–10 mg/dl acetocetic acid
• Blood	• 0.015–0.062 mg/dl hemoglobin
• Protein	• 15–30 mg/dl albumin

Glucose

The test is specific for glucose; no substance excreted in urine other than glucose is known to give a positive result. The reagent area does not react with lactose, galactose, fructose nor reducing metabolites of drugs (e.g., salicylates and nalidixic acic. This test may be used to determine whether the reducing substance found in urine is glucose. Reactivity may be influenced by urine specific gravity and temperature. In dilute urines containing less than 5 mg/dl ascorbic acid, as little as 40 mg/dl glucose may produce a color change that might be interpreted as positive. The test is more sensitive than the copper reduction test (e.g., CLINITEST® Reagent Tablets). If the color appears somewhat mottled at the higher glucose concentrations, match the darkest color to the color blocks.

Bilirubin

The test has a sensitivity of 0.4–0.8 mg/dL bilirubin.

Ketone

The test reacts with acetoacetic acid in urine. It does not react with acetone or 3-hydroxybutyric acid. Some high specific gravity/low pH urines may give reactions up to and including Trace. Clinical judgment is needed to determine the significance of reactions up to and including Trace.

Specific Gravity

The specific gravity test permits determination of urine specific gravity between 1.000 and 1.030. In general, it correlates within 0.005 with values obtained with the refractive index method. For increased accuracy, 0.005 may be added to readings from urines with pH equal to or greater than 6.5. Strips read instrumentally are automatically adjusted for pH by the instrument. The Bayer SG test is not affected by certain nonionic urine constituents such as glucose nor by the presence of radiopaque dye.

Blood

The sensitivity of this test may be reduced in urines with high specific gravity. The test is equally sensitive to myoglobin as to hemoglobin. The appearance of green spots on the reacted reagent area indicates the presence of intact erythrocytes in the urine. The Color Chart includes examples of Trace and moderate nonhemolyzed color blocks. Reactions ranging from Trace to large, with proportionately more numerous spots, may be observed (A hemoglobin concentration of 0.015–0.062 mg/dl is approximately equivalent to 5–20 intact red blood cells per microlitre). Because of the optical systems of urine chemistry instruments, the sensitivity to intact erythrocytes is lower than that perceived visually.

pH

The pH test area measures pH values generally to within 1 unit in the range of 5–8.5 visually and 5–9 instrumentally. pH readings are not affected by variations in the urinary buffer concentration.

Protein

The reagent area is more sensitive to albumin than to globulins, hemoglobin, Bence-Jones protein, and mucoprotein; a negative result does not rule out the presence of these other proteins.

Urobilinogen

This test area will detect urobilinogen in concentrations as low as 0.2 mg/dl (approximately 0.2 EU/dl) in urine. The absence of urobilinogen in the specimen cannot be determined.

Multistix® Urinalysis Strips (Fig. 5.2)

Dependable Results When and Where You Need Them

Bayer's Multistix strips lead the market in providing a range of rapid urine testing results. When read visually or automatically on either the Clinitek 50 or Clinitek 500 readers they enable on the spot clinical decisions to be made with confidence.

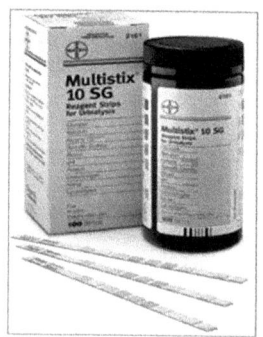

Fig. 5.2: Multistix® urinalysis strips.

Easy to Use (Figs. 5.3 to 5.5)

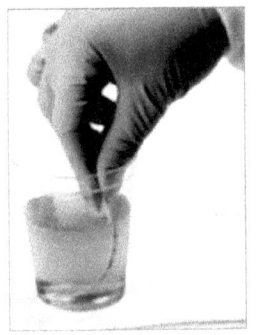

Fig. 5.3: Dip.

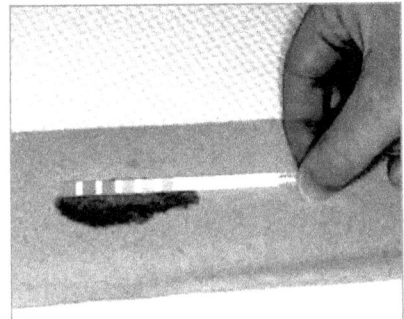

Fig. 5.4: Blot.

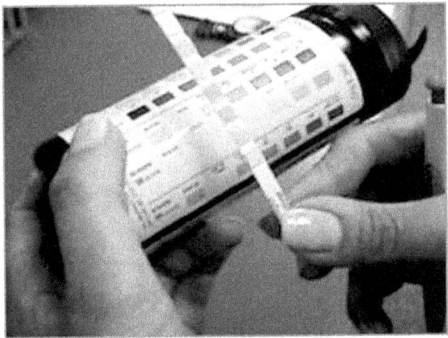

Fig. 5.5: Read at correct time.

Multistix Configurations

	Leuc	Nitrite	Urobil	Prot	pH	Blood	SG	Ket	Bill	Gluc
Multistix 10 SG	√	√	√	√	√	√	√	√	√	√
Multistix 8 SG	√	√		√	√	√	√	√		√
Multistix GP	√	√		√	√	√	√	√		√
N-Multistix SG		√	√	√	√	√	√	√	√	√
Multistix SG			√	√	√	√	√	√	√	√
Labstix SG				√	√	√	√	√		√
N-Labstix		√		√	√	√		√		√
Bili-Labstix				√	√	√		√	√	√
Labstix				√	√	√		√		√
Haema-Combistix				√	√	√				√
Uristix				√						√
Albustix				√						

Rapid Results

- Fast, reliable results available in 1-2 minutes
- Automated reading provided in 1 minute using.

First Line Health Screen for a Variety of Settings

Menu: Glucose, Ketones, Bilirubin, Urobilinogen, Specific Gravity, Blood, pH, Protein, Nitrite, Leucocytes.

Improved Use of Resources

- **Diabetes Management/Renal checks using microalbumin (Albumin : Creatinine Ratio) while the patient waits**
- Screens out non-infected urine samples so that only the positives need to be referred for laboratory follow-up in cases of Urinary Tract Infection.

STOOL EXAMINATION

Average healthy adults defecate from three times a day to three times a week. Common pattern is once a day. The stool tends to be soft and bulky on a diet high in vegetables and small and dry on a diet high in meat. Two thirds of the stool weight is attributable to its water content. The normal brown color is of still undetermined origin. The odor results from indole and skatole, produced by bacteria from tryptophan.

Feces are Composed of:

- Waste residue of indigestible material in food
- Bile (pigments and salts)
- Intestinal secretions, including mucus
- Leucocytes that migrate from the bloodstream
- Shed epithelial cells
- Large number of bacteria that make up to one-third of total solids

- Inorganic material (10–20%) that is chiefly calcium and phosphates
- Digested food (present in very small quantities).

Specimen Collection

A wide mouthed jar with a screw cap is good enough, provided it is neat, clean, and without any extraneous material in it. It should, however, never be overfilled and should be opened slowly to release the gas that accumulates frequently in it (if not done so, the contents may be released explosively). Since rectal evacuation is not completely at will and feces passed correlate very poorly with the food consumed; hence, collection should be done over a period of 3 days. The accuracy of this method can be enhanced somewhat by having the patient ingest carmine dye (0.3 g) and charcoal (1 g) at the beginning and the end of a collecting period, respectively, collecting the stools from the beginning of the appearance of the dye to the beginning of the appearance of the charcoal.

Be Careful

- Feces should be urine free when collected. Collect the entire stool and transfer to another container by a tongue blade. Deliver to the laboratory immediately after collection.
- Warm stools are best for detecting ova and parasites. Do not refrigerate for ova and parasites.
- Some coliform bacilli produce antibiotic substances that destroy enteric pathogens.
- Refrigerate stool if it cannot be examined immediately. Never place a stool in an incubator.
- A diarrheal stool will usually give good results.
- A freshly passed stool is the specimen of choice.

- Preferably, stool specimens should be collected before antibiotic therapy is initiated and as early in the course of disease as possible.
- Only a small amount of stool is needed; the size of a walnut. If mucus and blood are present, they should be included in part of the specimen to be examined.
- Do not use a stool that has been passed into the toilet bowl or that has been contaminated with barium or other X-ray medium.
- Label all stool specimens with patient's name, date, and reason for examination/testing.

Interfering Factors

- Meat interferes with some tests and should usually be omitted from the diet for 3 days before a test for blood (not necessary for the guaiac method)
- Stool specimens from patients receiving barium, bismuth, oil, or antibiotics are not satisfactory
- Bismuth from paper towels and toilet tissues interferes with tests.

Normal Values in Stool Analysis

See **Table 5.1.**

Inspection of Feces

A simple inspection of faeces may lead to a diagnosis of parasitic infection, obstructive jaundice, diarrhea, malabsorption, rectosigmoidal obstruction, dysentery or ulcerative colitis or gastrointestinal tract bleeding.

Note the quantity, form, consistency and color of the stool (**Table 5.2**).

Table 5.1: Normal values in stool analysis.

Macroscopic examination	Normal
Color	Brown
Odor	Varies with pH stool and depends upon bacterial fermentation and putrefaction
Consistency	Plastic; not unusual to see seeds and vegetable skins; soft and bulky in a high vegetable diet; small and dry in a high meat diet
Size and shape	Formed
Gross blood	Absent
Mucus	Absent
Pus	Absent
Parasites	Absent
Fat	Colorless, neutral fat (18%) and fatty acid crystals and soaps
Undigested	None to small amount food, meat fibers, starch, trypsin
Eggs and segments of parasites	Absent
Yeasts	Absent
Leucocytes	Absent
Chemical examination	Normal
pH	Neutral to weakly alkaline
Adult	7.0–7.5
Newborn	5.0–7.0

Contd...

Contd...

Macroscopic examination	Normal
Bottle-fed infants	Neutral to slightly alkaline pH of 7.0–8.0
Breast-fed infants	Slightly acidic
Occult blood	Negative
Urobilinogen	50–300 mg/24 hr
Porphyrins	Coproporphyrins < 200 µg/24 hr. Protoporphyrins < 1500 µg/24 hr. Uroporphyrins < 100 µg/24 hr.
Nitrogen	1–2 g/24 hr
Bile	Negative in adults, positive in children
Trypsin	Positive in small amounts in adults, in greater amounts in normal children.

Interfering Factors

- Stool darkens on standing
- Color is influenced by diet, food dyes, certain foods, and drugs.
    - Yellow to yellow green color occurs in the stool of breast-fed infants who lack normal intestinal flora. It also occurs in sterilization of bowel by antibiotic
    - Green color occurs in diets high in chlorophyll-rich vegetables and with use of the drug calomel
    - Black or very dark brown color may be due to drugs such as iron, charcoal, and bismuth, to foods such as cherries, or to an unusually high proportion of meat in the diet.
    - Light-colored stool with little odor may be due to diets high in milk and low in meat

Table 5.2: Inspection of feces.

Type of stool	Likely reason
Watery stool	Diarrhea
Large amount of mushy, foul smelling, gray stool that floats on water	Steatorrhea
Little firm, spherical masses	Constipation (irritable colon syndrome, overuse of laxatives)
Narrow ribbon-like stool	Spastic bowel or rectal narrowing or stricture
Clay colored	Obstructive jaundice or presence of Barium sulphate
Reddish stool	Blood from lower gastrointestinal tract, beets consumption or BSP use
Black, tarry stool	Bleeding from upper GIT, iron, bismuth or charcoal consumption
Green stool	Ingestion of spinach, etc., calomel, presence of biliverdin, seen in patients taking antibiotics orally
Parasites	Parasitic infestation (discussed later)

- Clay-like color may be due to a diet with excessive fat intake or barium used in X-ray examination
- Red color may be due to a diet high in beet or use of drugs such as BSP
- Drug-induced color changes are given below:
    » Black—iron salts, bismuth salts, charcoal
    » Green—mercurous chloride, indomethacin, calomel
    » Green to blue—dithiazanine

- » Brown staining—anthraquinones
- » Red—phenolphthalein, pyruvinium pamoate, tetracyclines in syrup, BSP
- » Yellow—santonin
- » Yellow to brown—senna
- » Light—sitosterols
- » Whitish discoloration—antacids
- » Orange red—phenazopyridine
- » Pink to red to black—anticoagulants (excessive dose) salicylates causing internal bleeding.

Pus

Patients with chronic ulcerative colitis and chronic bacillary dysentery frequently pass large quantities of pus with the stool that has to be examined microscopically.

It may also occur in localized abscesses or fistulas communicating with sigmoid rectum or anus. Large amounts of pus NEVER accompany amoebic colitis. No inflammatory exudate is seen in the watery stools of patients with viral gastroenteritis.

Mucus

Even in slightest quantity is abnormal (*see* **Table 5.3**).

Odor and pH

Normal Values

Characteristic odor varies with the pH of stool; normal pH is neutral or weakly alkaline.

The pH is dependent on bacterial fermentation and putrefaction in the bowel. Substances called indole and skatole, formed by

Table 5.3: Mucus in stool—causes.

Remarks	Causes
Translucent gelatinous mucus clinging to the surface of the formed stool.	Spastic constipation or mucus colitis. In emotionally disturbed patients and may result from excessive straining.
Bloody mucus clinging to stool mass.	Neoplasm, inflammation of rectal canal.
Mucus with pus and blood.	Ulcerative colitis, bacillary dysentery, ulcerating carcinoma of the colon, and more rarely, acute diverticulitis or intestinal tuberculosis.
Copious mucus, up to 3–4 litres of mucus per day.	Villous adenoma of the colon (may lead to dehydration and hypokalemia).

intestinal putrefaction and fermentation, are mainly responsible for the odor of normal stools.

Interfering Substances

Carbohydrate fermentation changes pH to acidic. Protein breakdown changes the pH to alkaline.

Blood

Blood in stools should never be ignored, however, slight the quantity may be. Bleeding in the upper GIT may give black-tarry appearance to stools while that arising from lower GIT may give red color or be seen as frank blood.

Causes

Upper GI Tract
- Peptic ulcer—gastric or duodenal
- Erosive gastritis
- Atrophic gastritis
- Esophageal varices
- Mallory-Weiss syndrome
- Hiatus hernia
- Esophagitis.

Small and Large Bowel
- Meckel's diverticulum
- Polyps
- Infectious diarrheas
- Inflammatory bowel disease (Crohn's disease, ulcerative colitis)
- Diverticular disease
- Vascular malformations
- Carcinoma.

Rectum and Anus
- Hemorrhoids
- Anorectal fissure.

Drugs
Associated with increased GIT blood loss.
- Salicylates
- Steroids
- Rauwolfia derivatives
- Indomethacin
- Colchicine.

Loss of more than 50–75 mL of blood from the upper GIT generally imparts a dark red to black color and a tarry consistency to the stool. Persistence of tarry appearance for two or three days suggests loss of at least 1000 mL of blood. Smaller increases in blood content may not alter appearance of the stool. Such stools are said to contain "*Occult Blood*" (usually associated with GIT neoplasm).

Interfering Factors

Drugs such as salicylates, steroids, indomethacin, colchicine, iron (used in massive therapy), and Rauwolfia derivatives are associated with increased gastrointestinal bleeding in normal persons and with even more pronounced bleeding when disease is present. Gastrointestinal bleeding tests may be falsely positive in the undermentioned circumstances:

- Meat in diet contains hemoglobin and enzymes that can give false-positive tests for up to 4 days after eating. The guaiac method does not require meat-free diet due to lesser sensitivity.
- Vitamin C taken in quantities greater than 500 mg per day may cause false-negative test for occult blood in stool.
- Drugs that may cause a false-positive test for occult blood include:
    - Boric acid   – Iodine
    - Bromides   – Inorganic iron
    - Colchicine   – Oxidizing agents
- Testing method must be followed exactly or the results are not reliable:
    - Use an aliquot from center of formed stool
    - Time reaction exactly
    - Liquid stools may cause false-negatives with filter paper methods.

Chapter 6: Body Fluids Analysis

CEREBROSPINAL AND OTHER BODY FLUIDS

CEREBROSPINAL FLUID

Cerebrospinal fluid (CSF) is formed primarily in ventricular choroid plexuses by a combination of both, active process and ultracentrifugation. Concentrations of sodium, chloride, magnesium and glutamine are greater in CSF than in plasma, while concentrations of glucose, potassium, calcium, cholesterol, uric acid, iron, thyroxine and zinc are lower in CSF.

Normal Values for Lumbar CSF in Adults

- Pressure   70–150 mm of water column (patient lying on side)
- Volume   90–150 ml
- Specific gravity   1.006–1.008
- Total solids   0.85–1.70 gm%
- Cells   0–8 lymphocytes/cu. mm
  Neutrophils and erythrocytes absent
- Protein   20–50 mg%

Of this
- albumin is 50-70%
- α_1 globulin is 3-9%
- α_2 globulin is 4-10%
- β globulin is 10-18%
- γ globulin is 3-9%
- fibrinogen is Absent

- Sodium 144-154 mEq/L
- Potassium 2.0-3.5 mEq/L
- Chloride 118-132 mEq/L
- pH 7.3-7.4
- Creatinine 0.5-1.2 mg%
- Cholesterol 0.2-0.6 mg%
- Glucose 50-80 mg%
- Glutamine 6-16 mg%
- Iron 1-2 mg%
- Thyroxine 0.1-0.2 mg%
- Urea 6-16 mg%
- Uric acid 0.5-4.5 mg%

Lumbar Puncture

Lumbar puncture needle is a long needle with a stylette inside. Lumbar puncture is usually performed at L3-L4 or lower to avoid damage to the spinal cord. In small children the conus medullaris extends lower than in adults, so puncture should be performed at L4-L5 or lower.

Indications

- Detection and diagnosis of suspected meningitis, subarachnoid hemorrhage, encephalitis, central nervous system (CNS) syphilis, spinal cord tumor or multiple sclerosis.

- Differential diagnosis of cerebral infarction vs intracerebral hemorrhage (almost 80% of latter show blood or xanthochromia)
- Introduction of anesthetics, radiographic contrast media or drugs
- Treatment of elevated CSF pressure in selected patients with benign intracranial hypertension
- Removal of exudate or blood from subarachnoid space.

The procedure should be done with a stylette inside to avoid implantation of skin which may form dermoid cyst in the spinal canal. A manometre and three-way stopcock should be attached to the needle, so that initial pressure can be accurately measured and CSF removed under control.

Complications of Lumbar Puncture

- Production of cerebellar pressure cone in patients with increased intracranial pressure.
- With spinal cord tumor, progression of paresis to paralysis may follow lumbar puncture.
- Introduction of infection by:
    - Passing the needle through superficial or deep sepsis in the lumbar region.
    - Improperly sterilized equipment.
    - Poor technique.
    - Development of dermoid cyst if lumbar puncture is performed without the stylette.
    - Postpuncture headache resulting from leakage of CSF (incidence can be decreased by using a small bore needle and keeping the patient horizontal for 24 hours).
- In infants death due to asphyxiation caused by restraint or tracheal obstruction from pushing the head forward.

Elective lumbar puncture should be performed in the morning rather than late afternoon or evening.

RISA injected into the lumbar subarachnoid space, the cotton is left in place for 12 hours and then counted for gamma radiation.

PLEURAL FLUID

The pleural surfaces are normally moistened by 1 to 10 ml of fluid derived by ultrafiltration of plasma. Normal protein concentration of this fluid is 1–2 gm% with no fibrinogen.

Pleural fluid parameter	Observation	SI units
Appearance	Clear, slightly amber	
Cholesterol		
Transudate	< 60 mg/dl	< 1.55 mmol/L
Exudate	> 60 mg/dl	> 1.55 mmol/L
Glucose		
Transudate	Approximates whole blood levels (whole blood adult normal 60–89 mg/dl, child normal 51–85 mg/dl)	
Exudate	Lower than whole blood levels	
Lactate dehydrogenase		
Transudate	< Client's serum LD (serum adult norm 45–90 U/L, child normal 60–170 U/L)	

Contd...

Contd...

Pleural fluid parameter	Observation	SI units
Exudate	> Client's serum LD	
pH	7.4	
Specific gravity		
Transudate	< 2.5 g/dl	<25 g/L
Exudate	> 3 g/dl	> 30 g/L
Volume	< 25 ml	
White blood cells		
Transudate	< 100/mm³	< 100 × 010⁹/L
Exudate	> 1000/mm³	> 1000 × 10⁹/L

Synovial Fluid Analysis

Synovial Analysis in Arthritis

	Appearance	Viscosity	White cells	Mucin clot	Protein total	(Avg-gm%) Globulin	Remarks
Normal	Straw-colored, clear, cloudy	High	200–600/25% poly's	Good	1.36	0.05	
Traumatic	Yellow to bloody	High	± 2000/30% poly's	Good	4.27		

Contd...

Contd...

	Appearance	Viscosity	White cells	Mucin clot	Protein total	(Avg-gm%) Globulin	Remarks
Osteoarthritis	Yellow, clear	High	± 1000/20% poly's	Good	3.08	0.75	Cartilage fibrils
Rheumatic	Yellow, slightly cloudy	Low	± 10,000/ 50% poly's	Good	3.74	1.07	
Systemic lupus erythematosus	Straw-colored, slightly cloudy	High	± 5000/10% poly's	Good			
Gout	Yellow to milky cloudy	Low	± 12,000/ 60% poly's	Fragile	4.18	1.54	Urate crystals
Tuberculous arthritis	Yellow, cloudy	Low	± 25,000 50–60% poly's	Fragile	5.3	2.0	Tubercle bacilli
Septic arthritis	Grayish or bloody, turbid	Low	± 80,000/ 90% poly's	Fragile	5.64	2.45	Bacteria
Rheumatoid arthritis	Yellow to greenish, cloudy	Low	± 15,000 65% ± poly's	Fragile	4.74	1.79	Rheumatoid factor

PERICARDIAL FLUID (PF)

The pericardial sac under normal circumstances contains 20–50 ml of clear, straw-colored fluid. A rapid abnormal accumulation of 200 ml may produce cardiac tamponade, while gradual accumulation of 1000 ml or more may be relatively asymptomatic.

Normal

Pericardial fluid parameter	Observation
Apperance	Clear to pale yellow
Glucose	
Transudate	Approximate whole blood levels (Whole blood adult norm 60–80 mg/dl, Whole blood child normal 51–85 mg/dl)
Exudate	Lower than whole blood levels
Lactate dehydrogenase	
Transudate	< Client's serum LD (serum adult normal 45–90 U/L, serum child normal 60–170 U/L)

PERITONEAL FLUID

Normally, the peritoneal cavity contains less than 100 ml of clear, straw-colored fluid.

Peritoneal fluid parameter	Observation	SI units
Appearance	Clear or pale yellow	
Albumin	Negative	

Contd...

Contd...

Peritoneal fluid parameter	Observation	SI units
Alkaline phosphatase		
Adult female	76–250 U/L	
Adult male	90–239 U/L	
Ammonia	< 50 gm/L	
Cholesterol		
Transudate	< 46 mg/dl	< 1.19 mmol/L
Exudate	> 46 mg/dl	> 1.19 mmol/L
Glucose transudate	60–100 mg/dl Lower than whole blood levels (Whole blood adult normal 60–89 mg/dl, child norm 51–85 mg/dl)	3.3–6.1 mmol/L
Lactic acid	10–20 mg/dl	1.1–2.3 mmol/L
Lactate dehydrogenase		
Transudate	< Client's serum LD (serum adult normal 45–90 U/L, child normal 60–170 U/L)	
Exudate	> Client's serum LD	
pH	7.4	

Contd...

Contd...

Peritoneal fluid parameter	Observation	SI units
Specific gravity		
Transudate	< 1.016	< 1.016
Exudate	> 1.016	> 1.016
Total protein		
Transudate	< 2.5 gm/dl	< 25 gm/L
Exudate	> 3 gm/dl	> 30 gm/L
Volume	< 100 ml	
White blood cells		
Transudate	< 100/mm^3	< 100 × 10^9/L
Exudate	> 1000/mm^3	> 1000 × 10^9/L

Indications for Abdominal Paracentesis

To be done under ultrasound guidance.
- Ascites of unknown etiology.
- Symptomatic ascites, e.g., dyspnea.
- Possible ruptured viscus or intra-abdominal hemorrhage due to trauma.
- Acute abdominal pain of unknown etiology.
- Postoperative hypotension and pain of unknown etiology.
- Instillation of cytotoxic drugs in ascites due to malignancy.

(The chief complication of abdominal paracentesis is intestinal perforation, perforation of other viscera is rare. If aspiration reveals gross blood or intestinal contents—laparotomy must be done).

AMNIOCENTESIS AND AMNIOTIC FLUID ANALYSIS, DIAGNOSTIC

Normal Value

Routine Analysis

Color: Colorless, straw-colored, or clear to milky.

Parameter	Observation	SI unit
Acetylcholinesterase	Negative	
Alpha1-fetoprotein		
12 weeks' gestation	<42 µg/ml	
14 weeks' gestation	<35 µg/ml	
16 weeks' gestation	<29 µg/ml	
18 weeks' gestation	<20 µg/ml	
20 weeks' gestation	<18 µg/ml	
22 weeks' gestation	<14 µg/ml	
30 weeks' gestation	<3 µg/ml	
35 weeks' gestation	<2 µg/ml	
40 weeks' gestation	<1 µg/ml	

Normal values may also be reported in multiples of the median (MOM) or 0.5–3.0 MOM.

Bilirubin

Trimester 1, 2	< 0.074 mg/dl	< 1.2 µmol/L
40 wks' gestation	< 0.024 mg/dl	<0.4 µmol/L
Calcium	4 mEq/L	4 mmol/L
Carbon dioxide	16 mEq/L	16 mmol/L
Chloride	102 mEq/L	102 mmol/L

Contd...

Contd...

Parameter	Observation	SI unit
Creatinine		
< 27 weeks' gestation	0.8–1.1 mg/dl	72–99 µmol/L
30–34 weeks' gestation	1.1–1.8 mg/dl	99–162 µmol/L
35–40 weeks' gestation	1.8–4.0 mg/dl	162–360 µmol/L
Estriol		
Trimester 1, 2	< 9 µg/dl	<309 µmol/L
Term	<59 ng/dl	<2023 µmol/L
Glucose	30 mg/dl	2 mmol/L
Lecithin		
<35 weeks' gestation	6–9 mg/dl	
> 35 weeks' gestation	15–20 mg/dl	
Lecithin/sphingomyelin (L/S)	Ratio	
Immaturity	< 1.5	
Borderline maturity	1.5–1.9	
Maturity	2.0–4.0	
Postmaturity	>4.1	
Meconium	Negative	
pH		
Trimester 1, 2	7.12–7.38	7.12–7.38
Term	6.91–7.43	6.91–7.43
Potassium	4.9 mEq/L	4.9 mmol/L
Sodium Sphingomyelin Total	133 mEq/L	133 mmol/L
Protein	4–6 mg/dl	
Urea	2.5 gm/dl	25 g/L

Contd...

Contd...

Parameter	Observation	SI unit
Trimester 1, 2	12–24 mg/dl	
Term	19–42 mg/dl	
Uric acid		
Trimester 1, 2	2.76–4.68 mg/dl	0.17–2.8 mmol/L
Term	7.67–12.13 mg/dl	0.46–0.72 mmol/L

Chapter 7

Sputum Examination

Tracheobronchial secretions are often collectively referred to as sputum. Sputum is constituted by plasma, water, electrolytes and mucin. As it comes out, it is contaminated by nasal and salivary secretions, and normal bacterial flora of the oral cavity. Under appropriate immunologic or inflammatory stimulus, mast cells, eosinophils and plasma cells may contribute to the secretions. Sputum is viscoelastic, i.e., some of the properties of a liquid. Chemical composition reveals sputum is 95% water and only 5% solids. The solid content increases with inflammation. It also shows exfoliation of lining cells.

SPECIMEN COLLECTION

- Before collecting or expectorating sputum, the mouth should be prerinsed and this removes contaminants from oral cavity especially.
- For most examinations, a first morning specimen is best as it represents the pulmonary secretions accumulated overnight.
- To obtain a good specimen, patient's cooperation and understanding is essential. Usually, no problem arises with adults. Children are problematic sometimes. The undermentioned methods can be used for them:

- A nasopharyngeal swab may be taken which is quite representative of the bronchial pathogens.
- A cough plate is held before the child's mouth and the child is urged to cough.
- Cough swab method gives the most representative, noncontaminated sputum sample. The child's mouth is held open by using a tongue depressor. Epiglottis is visualized and is touched with a swab to induce cough. Material expelled from trachea is (coughed) deposited on the swab, which can then be plated on appropriate culture media.
- In patients who are uncooperative or cannot produce adequate sputum, induction should be tried. Commonly used inductants are 10% sodium chloride, acetylcysteine and sterile or distilled water aerosols. In persons with a history of bronchospasmodic disorders, bronchodilators should be given after inductants are used. Acetylcysteine breaks the disulphide bonds which maintain the gel structure of mucus. Acetylcysteine can be given in an aerosol form with a bronchodilator.

The specimen should be collected in a sterile disposable, impermeable container with a screw cap.

SPUTUM EXAMINATION

Transfer the specimen in a sterile petridish placed against a dark background. Wooden applicator sticks can be used to spread it thinly and can be seen with the naked eye or by using a hand lens.

Macroscopic Examination

Volume: A 24-hour volume of sputum is measured in patients with chronic bronchitis, lung abscesses or bronchial asthma. A rising volume or decreasing volume indicates worsening and improvement respectively.

Consistency and Appearance

Sputum may be described as serous (liquid), mucoid, purulent, bloody or combinations of these, e.g., seropurulent, mucopurulent.

A normal sputum is clear and watery and any opalescence is because of cellular material suspended in it. In pulmonary edema sputum is serous, frothy and blood tinged. Most opaque particles are masses of pus and epithelium. Other materials seen in the sputum can be Curschmann's spirals, Dittrich's plugs, caseous material, bronchial casts, or food substances.

Color: Normal sputum is clear and colorless. A yellow color indicates pus and epithelial cells as seen in a pneumonic process.

Greenish tint implies *Pseudomonas* as the etiologic agent.

Rust colored sputum is due to decomposed hemoglobin and is seen in pneumococcal pneumonia or pulmonary gangrene, whereas a *bright red* sputum is found in recent hemorrhage which can follow acute cardiac infarction, pulmonary infarction, neoplasm invasion and rupture of a vessel.

Odor: Normal sputum is odorless. Suppurative pulmonary disorders such as lung abscesses, cavitary tuberculosis or gangrene produce most putrid odors. A ruptured subphrenic or liver abscess may impart a fecal odor.

Other Findings

- **Cheesy masses:** Fragments of necrotic pulmonary tissue seen in pulmonary gangrene or tuberculosis.

- **Bronchial casts:** These are branching tree-like casts of bronchi and their size depends upon the size of bronchi from which they have been expectorated. These can be seen in untreated lobar pneumonias, fibrinous bronchitis. To recognize these casts, they have to be floated on water against a black background.
- **Broncholiths (lung stones):** These are formed due to calcification of necrotic/infected tissue within a larger bronchus or cavity. The central core of these may be a foreign body or a fungus growth. Though rare, but when seen, chronic tuberculosis should be kept in mind.
- **Dittrich's plugs:** They are seen in putrid bronchitis and bronchiectasis. When expectorated, they are usually solitary of a variable size. When crushed, they are found to be made of cellular debris, fatty acid crystals, fat globules, and bacteria. These plugs are seen most commonly in chronic bronchitis, bronchiectasis and bronchial asthma.
- **Foreign bodies:** These are usually objects inhaled by a child. Usually, substances inhaled are peanuts and buttons. Radiologically, they are difficult to see.
- **Parasites:** Various parasites that can be seen in sputum are *Ascaris lumbricoides, Echinococcus granulosus, Toxocara canis* and *Paragonimus westermani*.

Chapter 8
Laboratory Investigations

HEMATOLOGY

Sl. No.	Determination No	Range Conventional units	SI units
1.	A$_2$ hemoglobin	2–3.2% of total Hb	Mass fraction 0.015–0.035 of total Hb
2.	Bleeding time	1.5–9.5 min	1.5–9.5 min
3.	Factor V assay (Proaccelerin factor)	60–140%	
4.	Factor VIII assay (Antihemophilic factor)	60–140%	
5.	Factor IX assay (plasma thromboplastin component)	60–140%	
6.	Factor X (Stuart factor)	60–140%	
7.	Fibrinogen	200–400 mg/dl	2–4 gm/dl

Contd...

Contd...

Sl. No.	Determination No	Range	
		Conventional units	SI units
8.	Fibrin split (degradation) products	< 5 µg/ml	< 5 µg/ml
9.	Partial thromboplastin time activated	20–25 sec lower limit 32–39 sec upper limit	
10.	Prothrombin consumption	10–14 sec	
11.	Prothrombin time	9.5–12 sec	
12.	INR In treatment	1 2.5–3 in AF, DVT, pulmonary embolism 2.5–3.5 for therapy in prosthetic heart valves	
13.	Erythrocyte count	**Males:** 4,600,000–6,200,000/cu.mm **Females:** 4,200,000–5,400,000/cu.mm	$4.6–6.2 \times 10^{12}/L$ $4.2–5.4 \times 10^{12}/L$
14.	Erythrocyte indices Mean corpuscular volume (MCV) Mean corpuscular Hb (MCH) Mean corpuscular Hb Concentration (MCHC) Reticulocytes	84–96 cu µm 28–33 µµg/cell 33–35% 0.5–1.5% of red cells	84–96 femtolitre 28–33 picogram Conc fraction 0.33–0.35 Number fraction 0.005–0.015

Contd...

Contd...

Sl. No.	Determination No	Range	
		Conventional units	SI units
15.	ESR (erythrocyte sedimentation rate) Westergren method	**Males:** < 50 years: < 15 mm/hr >50 years: < 20 mm/hr **Females:** < 50 years: < 25 mm/hr > 50 years: < 30 mm/hr	**Males:** < 50 years: < 15 mm/hr > 50 years: < 20 mm/hr **Females:** < 50 years: < 25 mm/hr > 50 years: < 30 mm/hr
16.	Erythrocyte sedimentation rate- Zeta centrifuge	<50 years: < 55% 50–80 years: 40–60%	Volume fraction: < 0.55 0.40–0.60
17.	Hematocrit	**Males:** 42–52% **Females:** 35–47%	Volume fraction: 0.42–0.52 Volume fraction: 0.35–47
18.	Hemoglobin	**Males:** 13–18 gm/dl **Females:** 12–16 gm/dl	2.02–2.79 mmol/L 1.86–2.48 mmol/L
19.	Hemoglobin F	< 2% of total Hb	Mass fraction: < 0.02
20.	Leukocyte alkaline phosphatase	15–30	

Contd...

Contd...

Sl. No.	Determination No	Range	
		Conventional units	SI units
21.	Leukocyte count	4,500–11,000/cu.mm	$4.5–11 \times 10^9$/L Number fraction
	Neutrophils	45–73%	0.45–0.73
	Eosinophils	0–4%	0.00–0.04
	Basophils	0–1%	0.00–0.01
	Lymphocytes	20–40%	0.20–0.40
	Monocytes	2–8%	0.02–0.08
22.	Platelet count	1,50,000–4,50,000/cu.mm	$0.15–0.45 \times 10^{12}$/L

SERUM, PLASMA AND WHOLE BLOOD CHEMISTRIES

Sl. No.	Determination	Range	
		Conventional units	SI units
1.	Acetoacetate	0.2–1 mg/dl	19.6–98 mmol/L
2.	Acetone	0.3–2 mg/dl	51.6–344 mmol/L
3.	Acid, total phosphatase	**Males:** 2–12 UL **Females:** 0.3–9.2 UL	2–12 UL 0.3–9.2 UL
4.	Acid, phosphatase Prostatic - RIA	2.5–3.37 ng/ml	2.5–3.37 µg/L
5.	Alkaline phosphate	Adults: 50–120 UL	50–120 UL
6.	Alkaline phosphatase Thermostable fraction	Hepatic : >25% Combined : 10–25% Skeletal : <10%	

Contd...

Contd...

Sl. No.	Determination	Range	
		Conventional units	SI units
7.	Adrenocorticotropic hormone (ACTH) Plasma- RIA	< 50 pg/ml	< 50 ng/ml
8.	Aldolase	3–8 Sibley–Lehninger U/dl at 37°C	22–59 mU/L at 37°C
9.	Aldosterone (plasma) RIA	Supine: 3–10 ng/d Upright: 5–30 ng/dl Adrenal vein: 200–800 ng/dl	0.08–0.30 nmol/L 0.14–0.90 nmol/L 5.54–22.16 nmol/L
10.	Alpha1 antitrypsin	110–140 mg/dl	1.1–1.4 gm/L
11.	Alpha 1 fetoprotein	< 15 ng/ml	< 15 µg/L
12.	Alpha hydroxybutyric dehydrogenase	< 140 U/L	< 2.33 µkat/L
13.	Ammonia (plasma)	15–45 µg/dl	11–32 µmol/L
14.	Amylase	60–160 somogyi U/dl	111–296 U/L
15.	Arsenic	< 70 µg/dl Poisoning:100–150 µg/dl	< 0.93–2.6 µmol/L 133–6.65 mmol/L
16.	Ascorbic acid	0.4–1.5 mg/dl	23–85 mmol/L
17.	Alanine aminotransferase (ALT) SGPT	**Males:** 10–40 U/L **Females:** 8–35 U/L	0.17–0.68 µkat/L 0.14–0.60 µkat/L

Contd...

Contd...

Sl. No.	Determination	Range Conventional units	SI units
18.	Aspartate aminotransferase AST (SGOT)	**Males:** 10–40 U/L **Females:** 15–30 U/L	0.34–0.68 µkat/L 0.25–0.51 µkat/L
19.	Bilirubin	Total: 0.3–1 mg/dl Direct: 0.1–0.4 mg/dl Indirect: 0.1–0.4 mg/dl	5–17 mmol/L 1.7–3.7 mmol/L 3.4–11.2 mmol/L
20.	Blood gases **(arterial)** Partial pressure of O_2 (PaO_2) SaO_2 CO_2 (PaCO_2) (whole blood) pH	85–95 mm Hg 95–99% 35–45 mm Hg 7.35–7.45	10.64–12.64 kPa Vol. Fraction 0.95–0.99 4.66–5.99 kPa 7.35–7.45
21.	Calcitonin stimulation test	**Basal:** <19 pg/ml **Males:** <350 pg/ml **Females:** <100 pg/ml	19 ng/L < 350 ng/L < 100 ng/L
22.	Calcium	8.6–10.2 mg/dl	2.15–2.55 mmol/L
23.	CO_2 venous	Adults: 24–32 mEq/L Infants: 18–24 mEq/L	24–32 mmol/L 18–24 mmol/L
24.	Catecholamines (plasma) RIA		
	Epinephrine	< 100 pg/ml	< 540 pmol/L
	Norepinephrine	< 400 pg/ml	< 2360 pmol/L
	Dopamine	< 143 pg/ml	< 935 pmol/L

Contd...

Contd...

Sl. No.	Determination	Range Conventional units	SI units
25.	Ceruloplasmin	20–40 mg/dl	1.26–2.52 mmol/L
26.	Chloride	97–107 mEq/L	97–107 mmol/L
27.	Cholesterol	150–200 mg/dl	3.9–5.2 mmol/L
28.	Cholesterol esters	60–70% of total cholesterol	Fraction of total cholesterol 0.6–0.7
29.	Cholinesterase	Serum: 0.6–1.6 delta pH	0.6–1.6 U
		Red cells: 0.6–1 delta pH	0.6–1 U
30.	Chorionic gonadotropin Beta subunit	0–5 IU/L	0–5 IU/L
31.	Complement C_3	80–170 mg/dl	0.8–1.7 gm/L
32.	Complement C_4	18–51 mg/dl	180–510 mg/L
33.	Complement total hemolytic	90–94% complement	27–70 U/ml
34.	Copper	75–150 µg/dl	11–24 µmol/L
35.	Cortisol-RIA	**8 am:** 5–25 µg/dl **4 pm:** 3–16 µg/dl	138–690 nmol/L 83–442 nmol/L

Contd...

Contd...

Sl. No.	Determination	Range Conventional units	SI units
36.	C-peptide reactivity	0.9–4 ng/ml	0.9–4 µg/L
37.	Creatine	0.2–0.8 mg/L	15.3–61 µmol/L
38.	Creatine phosphokinase	**Males:** 50–325 mU/ml **Females:** 50–250 mU/ml	50–325 U/L 50–250 U/L
39.	Creatine phosphokinase isoenzymes	MM+ skeletal muscle MB absent heart muscle	
40.	Creatinine	0.7–1.4 mg/dl	62–124 µmol/L
41.	Creatinine clearance	**Males:** 85–125 ml/min **Females:** 75–115 ml/min	1.42–2.08 ml/s 1.25–1.92 ml/s
42.	Cryoglobins, qualitative	Negative	
43.	11- Deoxycortisol	1 µg/dl	< 0.029 µmol/L
44.	Dibucaine number	Normal: 70–85% inhibition Heterozygote: 50–65% inhibition Homozygote: 16–25% inhibition	
45.	Dihydrotestosterone	**Males:** 50–210 ng/dl **Females:** None	1.72–7.22 nmol/L

Contd...

Contd...

Sl. No.	Determination	Range	
		Conventional units	SI units
46.	Estradiol- RIA	**Females:**	
		Follicular: 10–90 pg/ml	37–370 pmol/L
		Midcycle: 100–500 pg/ml	367–1835 pmol/L
		Luteal: 50–240 pg/ml	184–881 pmol/L
		Follicular phase: 2–20 ng/dl	
		Midcycle: 12–40 ng/dl	
		Luteal phase: 10–30 ng/dl	
		Postmenopausal: 1–5 ng/dl	
		Males: 0.5–5 ng/dl	
47.	Estriol –RIA	**Nonpregnant females:** < 0.5 ng/ml	< 1.75 nmol/L
		Pregnant females: 1st trimester: Upto 1 ng/ml	Upto 3.5 nmol/L
		2nd trimester: 0.8–7 ng/ml	2.8–24.3 nmol/L
		3rd trimester: 5–25 ng/ml	17.4–86.8 nmol/L
48.	Estrogens, total RIA	**Females: Cycle days**	
		Day 1–10: 61–394 pg/ml	61–394 ng/L
		Day 11–20: 122–437 pg/ml	122–437 ng/L
		Day 21–30: 156–350 pg/ml	156–350 ng/L
		Males: 40–115 pg/ml	40–115 ng/L

Contd...

Contd...

Sl. No.	Determination	Range	
		Conventional units	SI units
49.	Estrone–RIA	**Females:**	
		Day 1–10: 4.3–18 ng/dl	15.9–66.6 pmol/lL
		Day 11–20 : 7.5–19.6 ng/dl	27.8–72.5 pmol/L
		Day 21–30: 13–20 ng/dl	48.1–74 pmol/L
		Males: 2.5–7.5 ng/ml	9.3–27.8 pmol/L
50.	Ferritin–RIA	**Males:** 20–250 ng/ml	20–250 µg/L
		Females: 12–250 ng/ml	12–250 µg/L ng/ml
51.	Folic acid- RIA	2.5–20 ng/ml	6–46 nmol/L
52.	Follicle stimulating hormone (FSH)- RIA	**Males:** 2–10 mIU/ml	
		Females:	
		Follicular phase: 5–20 mIU/ml	5–20 IU/L
		Peak of middle cycle: 12–30 mIU/ml	12–30 IU/L
		Luteinic phase: 5–15 mIU/ml	5–15 IU/L
		Menopausal females:	
		40–200 mIU/ml	40–200 IU/L
53.	Galactose	< 5 mg/dl	< 0.28 mmol/L
54.	Gamma glutamyl transpeptidase	**Males:** 20–30 U/L	0.03–0.5 µkat/L
		Females: 1–24 U/L	0.02–0.4 µkat/L
55.	Gastrin –RIA	**Fasting:** 50–155 pg/ml	50–155 ng/L
		Postprandial:	
		80–170 pg/ml	80–170 ng/L

Contd...

Contd...

Sl. No.	Determination	Range	
		Conventional units	SI units
56.	Glucose	**Fasting:** 60–110 mg/dl **Postprandial 2 hr:** 65–140 mg/dl	3.3–6.05 mmol/L 3.58–7.7 mmol/L
57.	Glucose tolerance	**Normal fasting:** 60–110 mg/dl No sugar in urine Upper limits of Normal: Fasting: 125 mg/dl 1 hr 190 mg/dl 2 hrs 140 mg/dl 3 hrs 125 mg/dl	3.3–6.05 mmol/L 6.88 mmol/L 10.45 mmol/L 7.7 mmol/L 6.88 mmol/L
58.	Glucose 6 phosphate dehydrogenase (red cells)	**Screening:** Decolorization: 20–100 mts **Quantitative:** 1.86–2.5 IU/ml RBC	1860–2500 U/L
59.	Glycoprotein Alpha-1–acid	50–120 mg/dl	0.5–1.2 gm/L
60.	Growth hormone RIA	**Males:** 0–4 ng/ml **Females:** 0–18 ng/ml	0.4 µg/L 0–18 µg/L
61.	Haptoglobin	30–200 mg/dl	0.3–2 gm/L
62.	Hemoglobin plasma	0.5–5 mg/dl	5–50 mg/L

Contd...

Contd...

Sl. No.	Determination	Range	
		Conventional units	SI units
63.	Glycohemoglobin (GHB, hemoglobin A$_{1c}$, HbA1)	Non-diabetics and diabetics with good control 4.4%–6.4%	
63A.	Hexosaminidase total	**Controls:** 333–375 nM/ml/h	333–375 µmol/L/h
64.	High density lipoprotein cholesterol (HDL)	**Males:** 35–70 mg/dl **Females:** 35–85 mg/dl	0.91–1.81 mmol/L 0.91–2.20 mmol/L
65.	17- hydroxyl progesterone- RIA	**Males:** 0.5–2 ng/ml **Females:** 0.2–3 ng/ml **Children:** <1 ng/ml	1.5–6 nmol/L 0.6–9 nmol/L < 3 nmol/L
66.	Immunoglobulin A	Adults: 85–385 mg/dl Varies with age, low in children	0.85–3.85 gm/L
67.	Immunoglobulin D	0–14 mg/dl	0–140 mg/L
68.	Immunoglobulin E	100–700 ng/ml	100–700 µg/L
69.	Immunoglobulin G	Adults: 565–1765 mg/dl	6.35–14 gm/L
70.	Immunoglobulin M	Adults : 55– 375 mg/dl	0.4–2.8 gm/L
71.	Insulin–RIA	5–25 µU/ml	0.2–1 µg/L
72.	Iron	50–160 µg/dl	9–29 µmol/L
73.	Iron binding capacity	IBC: 250–350 µg/dl TIBC: 250–475 µg/dl % saturation: 20–50	45–63 µmol/L 45–85 µmol/L Fraction of TIBC 0.2–0.5

Contd...

Contd...

Sl. No.	Determination	Range Conventional units	SI units
74.	Isocitric dehydrogenase	50–180 U	0.83–3 UIL
75.	Lactic acid (whole blood)	Venous: 5–15 mg/dl Arterial: 3–11 mg/dl	0.5–1.7 mmol/L 0.36–1.25 mmol/L
76.	Lactic dehydrogenase (LDH)	90–176 mU/ml	90–176 U/L
77.	LDH isoenzymes		
	Total LDH		
	LDH 1	22–36%	0.2–0.36
	LDH 2	35–46%	0.35–0.46
	LDH 3	13–26%	0.13–0.26
	LDH 4	3–10%	0.03–0.10
	LDH 5	2–12%	0.02–0.12
78.	Lead (whole blood)	Upto 40 µg/dl	Upto 2 µmol/L
79.	Leucine aminopeptidase	80–200 U/ml	19.2–48 U/L
80.	Lipase	< 200 U/ml	< 200 U/L
81.	Lipids total	400–800 mg/dl	4–8 gm/L
82.	LDL cholesterol	< 160 mg/dl if no CAD < 130 mg/dl if no CAD +2 or more risk factors < 100 mg/dl if CAD +	

Contd...

Contd...

Sl. No.	Determination	Range	
		Conventional units	SI units
83	Luteinizing hormone –RIA	**Males:** 1.5–9.3 mU/ml **Females:** Follicular phase: 1.9–12.5 mU/ml Midcycle: 8.7–76.3 mU/ml	1.5–9.3 U/L 1.9–12.5 U/L 8.7–76.3 U/L
84.	Lysozyme (muramidase)	4–15.6 µg/ml	0.28–1.10 µmol/L
85.	Magnesium	1.3–2.3 mg/dl	0.62–0.95 mmol/L
86.	Mercury	< 10 µg/L	< 50 µmol/L
87.	Myoglobin-RIA	5–70 ng/ml	5–70 µg/ml
88.	5 nucleotidase	3.2–11.6 IU/L	3.2–11.6 U/L
89.	Osmolality	275–300 mOsm/kg	275–300 mmol/L
90.	Parathyroid hormone	10–65 pg/ml	10–65 ng/L
91.	Phenylalanine	1.2–3.5 mg/dl 1st week	0.07–0.21 mmol/L
		0.7 -3.5 mg/dl thereafter	0.04–0.21 mmol/L
92.	Phosphohexose isomerase	20–90 IU/L	20–90 U/L
93.	Phospholipids	125–300 mg/dl	1.25–3 g/L
94.	Phosphorus inorganic	2.5–4.5 mg/dl	0.8–1.45 mmol/L
95.	Potassium	3.5–5 mEq/L	3.5–5 mmol/L

Contd...

Contd...

Sl. No.	Determination	Range	
		Conventional units	*SI units*
96.	Progesterone–RIA	Follicular phase upto 0.8 ng/ml	2.5 nmol/L
		Luteal phase: 10–20 ng/ml	31.8–63.6 nmol/L
		End of cycle: <1 ng/ml	< 3 nmol/L
		Pregnant: Upto 50 ng/ml in 20th wk	Upto 160 nmol/L
97.	Prolactin–RIA	4–30 ng/ml	4–30 µg/ml
98.	Prostate–specific antigen	< 4 ng/ml	
99.	Protein–total Albumin Globulin	6–8 gm/dl 4–5.5 gm/dl 1.7–3.3 gm/dl	60–80 gm/L 40–55 gm/L 17–33 gm/L
100.	Protein Electrophoresis	35–50 gm/L	
	Albumin	4.0–5.5 gm/dl	40–55 gm/L
	Alpha-1-globuln	0.15–0.25 gm/dl	1.5–2.5 gm/L
	Alpha-2–globulin	0.43–0.75 gm/dl	4.3–7.5 gm/L
	Beta globulin	0.5–1.0 gm/dl	5–10 gm/L
	Gamma gobulin	0.6–1.3 gm/dl	6–13 gm/L
101.	Protoporphyrin erythrocyte (whole blood)	**Males:** 11–45 µg/dl **Females:** 19–52 µg/dl	0.20–0.8 µmol/L 0.34–0.92 µmol/L

Contd...

Contd...

Sl. No.	Determination	Range	
		Conventional units	SI units
102.	Pyridoxine	5–30 ng/ml	20–1.21 nmol/L
103.	Pyruvic acid (whole blood)	0.3–0.9 mg/dl	34–102 µmol/L
104.	Renin (plasma)	Normal diet supine: 0.3–1.9 ng/ml/hr	0.08–0.52 ng/L/S
		Upright: 0.6–3.6 ng/ml/hr	0.16–1.00 µg/L/S
		Low salt diet: Supine: 0.9–4.5 ng/ml/hr	0.25–1.25 µg/L/S
		Upright: 4.1–9.1 ng/ml/hr	1.13–2.53 µg/L/S
105.	Sodium	135–145 mEq/L	135–145 mmol/L
106.	Sulphate inorganic	0.5–1.5 mg/dl	0.05–0.15 mmol/L
107.	Testosterone–RIA	**Females:** 20–80 ng/dl	0.7–2.8 nmol/L
		Males: 240–1200 ng/dl	18.3–41.8 nmol/L
108.	T3 Triiodothyronine Uptake	24–34%	Relative uptake fraction: 0.24–0.34
109.	T3 total circulating RIA	70–204 ng/dl	1.08–3.14 nmol/L
110.	T4 Thyroxine RIA	5–11 µg/dl	65–138 nmol/L
111.	T4 free	0.8–2.7 ng/dl	10.3–35 pmol/L
112.	Thyroid stimulating hormone TSH-RIA		0.4–4.2 mIU/L

Contd...

Contd...

Sl. No.	Determination	Range Conventional units	SI units
113.	Thyroid binding globulin	10–26 µg/dl	100–260 µg/L
114.	Transferrin	200–380 mg/dl	2.3–3.2 gm/L
115.	Triglycerides	100–200 mg/dl	1.13–3.8 mmol/L
116.	Tryptophan	1.4–3 mg/dl	68.6–147 nmol/L
117.	Tyrosine	0.5–4 mg/dl	27.6–220.8 mmol/L
118.	Urea nitrogen (BUN)	10–20 mg/dl	3.6–7.2 mmol/L
119.	Uric acid	2.5–8 mg/dl	0.15–0.5 mmol/L
120.	Viscosity	1.4–1.8 relative to water at 37°C	
121.	Vitamin A	30–120 µg/dl	1.05–4.20 µmol/L
122.	Vitamin B (Thiamine)	1.6–4 µg/dl	47.4–135.7 nmol/L
123.	Vitamin B_6 (pyridoxal phosphate)	5–30 ng/ml	20–121 nmol/L
124.	Vitamin B_{12}–RIA	200–900 pg/ml	148–666 pmol/L
125.	Vitamin E	0.5–1.8 mg/dl	12–42 µmol/L
126.	Xylose absorption test	2 hr: 30–50 mg/dl	2–3.35 mmol/L
127.	Zinc	55–150 µg/dl	7.65–22.95 µmol/L

URINE CHEMISTRY

Sl. No.	Determination	Normal ranges — Conventional units	SI units
1.	Acetone and acetoacetate	Zero	
2.	Acid mucopolysaccharides	Negative	
3.	Aldosterone	**With normal salt diet:** Normal: 4–20 µg/24 h Renovascular: 10–40 µg/24 h Tumor: 20–100 µg/24 h	11.1–55.5 nmol 27.7–111 nmol/24 h 55.4–277 nmol/24 h
4.	Alpha amino nitrogen	50–200 mg/24 h	3.6–14.3 nmol/24 h
5.	Amylase	35–260 urine excreted/hour	6.5–48.1 U/h
6.	Arylsulfatase A	> 2.4 units/ml	
7.	Bence-Jones protein	None detected	
8.	Calcium	< 150 mg/24 hrs	2.5–6.2 mmol/24 hrs
9.	Catecholamines	Total: 0–275 µg/24 hrs Epinephrine: 10–40% Norepinephrine: 60–90%	0–275 µg/24 hrs Fraction total: 0.10–8.4 Fraction total: 0.60–0.90

Contd...

Contd...

Sl. No.	Determination	Normal ranges — Conventional units	SI units
10.	Chorionic gonadotropin, qualitative (pregnancy test)	Negative	
11.	Copper	15–60 µg/24 hrs	0.22–0.9 µmol/24 hrs
12.	Coproporphyrin	50–300 µg/24 hrs	0.075–0.45 µmol/24 hrs
13.	Cortisol free	20–90 µg/24 hrs	55.2–248.4 nmol/day
14.	Creatinine	**Males:** 1–2 gm/24 hrs	8.8–17.7 mmol/24 hrs
		Females: 0.8–1.8 gm/24 hrs	7.1–15.9 mmol/24 hrs
15.	Creatine	0–270 mg/24 hrs	0–2.05 mmol/24 hrs
16.	Creatinine clearance	**Males:** 85–125 ml/min	1.42–2.08 ml/s
		Females: 75–115 ml/min	1.25–1.92 ml/s
17.	Cystine and cysteine	10–100 mg/24 hrs	0.08–0.83 mmol/24 hrs
18.	Delta aminolevulinic acid	0.00–0.54 mg/dl	0–40 µmol/l
19.	11-Deoxycortisol	20–100 µg/24 hrs	0.6–32.9 µmol/day

Contd...

Contd...

Sl. No.	Determination	Normal ranges	
		Conventional units	SI units
20.	Estriol (placental)	Wks of pregnancy / μm/24 hr / mmol/24 hr 12 <1 <3.5 16 2–7 7–24.5 20 4–9 14–32 24 6–13 21–45.5 28 8–22 28–77 32 12–43 42–150 36 14–45 49–158 40 19–46 66.5–160	
21.	Estrogens, total (fluorometric)	**Females:** Onset of menstruation: 4–25 μg/24 hrs Ovulation peak: 28–100 μg/24 hrs Luteal peak: 22–105 μg/24 hrs **Menopausal:** 1.4–19.6 μg/24 hrs **Males:** 5–18 μg/24 hrs	4–25 μg/24 hrs 28–100 μg/24 hrs 22–105 μg/24 hrs 1.4–19.6 μg/24 hrs 5–18 μg/24 hrs

Contd...

Contd...

Sl. No.	Determination	Normal ranges	
		Conventional units	**SI units**
22.	Etiocholanolone	**Males:** 1.9–6 mg/24 hrs **Females:** 0.5–4 mg/24 hrs	6.5–20.6 µmol/24 hrs 1.7–13.8 µmol/24 hrs
23.	Follicle stimulating hormone -RIA	**Females:** **Follicular:** 5–20 IU/24 hrs **Luteal:** 5–15 IU/24 hrs **Midcycle:** 15–60 IU/24 hrs **Menopausal:** 50–100 IU/24 hrs **Males:** 5–25 IU/24 hrs	5–20 IU/day 5–15 IU/day 15–60 IU/day 50–100 IU/day 5–25 IU/day
24.	Glucose	Negative	
25.	Hemoglobin and myoglobin	Negative	
26.	Homovanillic acid		< 44 µmol/24 hrs
27.	17 hydroxy-corticosteroids	8 mg/24 hrs 2–10 mg/24 hrs	5.5–27.5 µmol/day
28.	Hydroxyproline	25–77 mg/24 hrs	
29.	5 hydroxyindoleacetic acid, qualitative	Negative	
30.	17- ketosteroids, total	**Males:** 10–22 mg/24 hrs **Females:** 6–16 mg/24 hrs	35–76 µmol/24 hrs 21–55 µmol/24 hrs
31.	Kyurenic and xanthurenic acids	**Kyurenic acid:** Upto 18 mg/24 hrs **Xanthurenic acid:** Upto 4 mg/24 hrs	

Contd...

Contd...

Sl. No.	Determination	Normal ranges	
		Conventional units	SI units
32.	Lead	< 125 µg/24 hrs	< 60 µmol/24 hrs
33.	Luteinizing hormone	**Males:** 5–18 IU/24 hrs **Females:** **Follicular phase:** 2–25 IU/24 hrs **Ovulatory phase:** 30–95 IU/24 hrs **Luteal phase:** 2–20 IU/24 hrs **Postmenopausal:** 40–110 IU/24 hrs	2–25 IU/day 30–95 IU/day 2–20 IU/day 40–110 IU/day
34.	Metanephrines, total	< 1.4 mg/24 hrs	< 7 µmol/24 hrs
35.	Osmolality	250–900 mOsm/kg	250–900 mmol/kg
36.	Oxalate	Upto 45 mg/24 hrs	Upto 500 µmol/24 hrs
37.	Phenylpyruvic acid	Negative	
38.	Phosphorus, inorganic	0.9–1.3 gm/24 hrs	29–42 mmol/24 hrs
39.	Porphobilinogen, qualitative	Negative	
40.	Porphobilinogen, quantitative	0–1 mg/24 hrs	0–4.4 µmol/24 hrs
41.	Porphyrins, qualitative	Negative	

Contd...

Contd...

Sl. No.	Determination	Normal ranges	
		Conventional units	**SI units**
42.	Porphyrins, quantitative	**Coproporphyrin:** 50–160 µg/24 hrs **Uroporphyrin:** upto 50 µg/24 hrs	0.075–0.24 µmol/24 hrs upto 0.06 µmol/24 hrs
43.	Potassium	40–65 mEq/24 hrs	26–123 mmol/24 hrs
44.	Pregnanediol	**Females:** **Proliferative phase:** 0.5–1.5 mg/24 hrs	1.6–4.8 µmol/24 hrs
		Luteal phase: 2–7 mg/24 hrs **Menopause:** 0.2–1 mg/24 hrs Pregnancy: Weeks of mg/ **Gestation** 24 hrs 10–12 5–15 12–18 5–25 18–24 15–33 24–28 20–42 28–32 27–47	6–22 µmol/24 hrs 0.6–3.1 µmol/24 hrs µmol/24 hrs 15.6–47 15.6–78 47–103 62.4–131 84.2–146.6
45.	Pregnanetriol	**Females:** 0.1–2.2 mg/24 hrs **Males:** 0.4–2.5 mg/24 hrs	0.3–6.5 µmol/24 hrs 1.2–7.5 µmol/24 hrs
46.	Protein	< 150 mg/24 hrs	< 150 mg/24 hrs
47.	Sodium	75–200 mEq/24 hrs	75–200 mmol/24 hrs

Contd...

Contd...

Sl. No.	Determination	Normal ranges	
		Conventional units	SI units
48.	Titratable acidity	20–40 mEq/2 hrs	20–40 mmol/24 hrs
49.	Urea nitrogen	9–16 gm/24 hrs	0.32–0.57 mmol/L
50.	Uric acid	250–750 mg/24 hrs	1.48–4.43 mmol/24 hrs
51.	Urobilinogen	**Random urine:** <0.25 mg/dl 24 hr urine: upto 4 mg/24 hrs	< 0.42 mol/24 hrs upto 6.76 µmol/24 hrs
52.	Uroporphyrins	Upto 50 µg/24 hrs	
53.	Vanillylmandelic acid (VMA)	0.7–0.8 mg/24 hrs	3.5–34.3 µmol/24 hrs
54.	Xylose absorption test (5 hours)	16–33% of ingested xylose	Fraction absorbed: 0.16–0.33
55.	Zinc	0.15–1.2 mg/24 hrs	2.3–18.4 µmol/24 hrs

IMMUNODIAGNOSTIC TEST

Sl. No.	Determination	Normal value
1.	Acetylcholine receptor binding antibody	Negative or < 0.03 nmol/L
2.	Anti-ls-DNA antibody	<70 U by ELISA <1:20 by indirect fluorescence

Contd...

Contd...

Sl. No.	Determination	Normal value
3.	Anti-glomerular basement membrane antibody	Negative or < 5 EU/ml
4.	Anti-insulin antibody	< 3% binding of labelled beef and pork insulin by patient's serum or <9 ml/m IU/L
5.	Antinuclear antibody	Negative, <1:40
6.	Anti parietal cell antibody	Negative
7.	Antiribonucleoprotein antibody	Negative
8.	Antiscleroderma	Negative
9.	Anti-Smith antibody	Negative
10.	Anti-SS-A/anti-SS-B	Negative
11.	Antithyroglobulin and antimicrosomal antibodies	<1:100 titer by gelatin or hemagglutination
12.	CA 15–3 tumor marker	< 30 IU/ml
13.	CA 19–9 tumor marker	< 37 IU/ml
14.	CA 125	0–35 IU/ml
15.	Carcinoembryonic Antigen (CEA)-RLK	0–2.5 µg/L (non-smoker) 0–5 µg/L (smoker)
16.	Cold agglutinins	Negative or <1:32
17.	C-reactive protein	< 0.8 mg/dl
18.	Cytomegalovirus antibodies (CMV IgM)	Negative < 0.9 units/ml

Contd...

Contd...

Sl. No.	Determination	Normal value
19.	Cytomegalovirus (CMV IgM)	Negative: < 0:79 Equivocal: 0:80–1.20
20.	Epstein-Barr virus serology (viral capsid antigen IgG and Ig M, early antigen IgG and nuclear antigen IgG)	Negative: <1:20 or < 1:20 for each individual test
21.	Hepatitis A virus antibodies IgM (HAV- Ab/IgM)	Negative
22.	Hepatitis A virus antibodies IgG (HAV-Ab/IgG)	Negative
23.	Hepatitis B surface antigen (HBs Ag)	Negative
24.	Hepatitis B surface antibody (HBsAb)	Negative
25.	Hepatitis C virus antibodies	Negative
26.	Hepatitis C virus RNA	Negative
27.	Infectious mononucleosis tests (monospot, mono test, heterophile antigen test, Epstein-Barr virus EBV)	Negative
28.	Lyme disease titer	Negative, <1:256 by indirect fluorescent antibody method: nonreactive by ELISA
29.	Pyroglobulin test Rheumatoid factor	Negative or < 40 IU/ml

Contd...

Contd...

Sl. No.	Determination	Normal value
30.	T and B cell lymphocyte surface markers T-helper/T-suppressor ratio	**T and B cell lymphocyte surface markers:** Percent T cells (CD 2): 60–88% Percent helper cells (CD4): 34–67% Percent suppressor cells (CD 8): 10–42% Percent B cells (CD 19): 3–21% **Absolute counts:** Lymphocyte: 0.66–4.60 thousand/ml T cells: 644–2201 cells/ml Helper cells: 493–1191 cells/ml Suppressor: T cells: 182–785 cells/ml B cells: 92–392 cells/ml Lymphocyte ratio: TH/TS ratio >1

CEREBROSPINAL FLUID

Sl. No.	Determination	Normal value
1.	Albumin	15.5–32 mg/dl
2.	Cell count	0–5 mononuclear cells/cu.mm
3.	Chloride	100–130 mEq/L
4.	Glucose	50–75 mg/dl
5.	Glutamine	6–15 mg/dl

Contd...

Contd...

Sl. No.	Determination	Normal value
6.	IgG	0–6.6 mg/dl
7.	Lactic acid	< 24 mg/dl
8.	Lactic dehydrogenase	One tenth that of serum
9.	Protein lumbar cisternal ventricular	15–45 mg/dl 15–25 mg/dl 5–15 mg/dl
10.	Protein electrophoresis Prealbumin Albumin Alpha 1 globulin Alpha 2 globulin Beta globulin Gamma globulin	% of total protein: 3–7 56–74 2–6.5 3–12 8–18.5 4–14

MISCELLANEOUS VALUES

Therapeutic Levels

Sl. No.	Determination	Normal value	Clinical significance
1.	Acetaminophen	Zero	Therapeutic level: 10–20 µg/ml
2.	Aminophylline	Zero	Therapeutic level: 10–20 µg/ml
3.	Bromide	Zero	Therapeutic level: 5–50 mg/dl
4.	Carbamazepine	Zero	Therapeutic level: 8–12 µg/ml
5.	Carbon monoxide	0–2%	Symptoms with over 20%
6.	Chlordiazepoxide	Zero	Therapeutic level: 1–3 µg/ml
7.	Diazepam	Zero	Therapeutic level: 0.5–2.5 µg/dl

Contd...

Contd...

Sl. No.	Determination	Normal value	Clinical significance
8.	Digitoxin	Zero	5–30 ng/ml
9.	Digoxin	Zero	Therapeutic level: 0.5–2 ng/ml
10.	Ethanol	0–0.1%	Legal intoxication level: 0.10% or above 0.3–0.4 %= marked intoxication 0.4–0.5 %= alcoholic stupor
11.	Gentamicin	Zero	Therapeutic level: 15–40 µg/ml
12.	Lithium	Zero	Therapeutic level: 0.6–1.2 mEq/l
13.	Methanol	Zero	May be fatal in concentrations as low as 10 mg/dl
14.	Phenobarbital	Zero	Therapeutic level: 15–40 µg/ml
15.	Phenytoin	Zero	Therapeutic level: 10–20 µg/ml
16.	Primidone	Zero	Therapeutic level: 5–12 µg/ml
17.	Quinidine	Zero	Therapeutic level: 0.2–0.5 mg/dl
18.	Salicylate	Zero	Therapeutic level: 2–25 mg/dl Toxic level: > 30 mg/dl
19.	Sulfonamide	Zero	Therapeutic levels: Sulfadiazine 8–15 mg/dl Sulfaguanidine 3–5 mg/dl Sulfamerazine 10–15 mg/dl Sulphanilamide 10–15 mg/dl
20.	Vancomycin	Zero	Therapeutic level peak: 20–40 µg/ml Therapeutic trough: 5–10 µg/ml

Gastric Analysis

Gastric analysis	Normal value	Increased	Decreased
pH	< 2		Pernicious anaemia
Basal acid output	0–6 mEq/hr	Peptic ulcer	Gastric carcinoma
Maximum acid	5–40 mEq/hr	Zollinger-Ellison syndrome	Chronic atopic gastritis Decreased normally with age

Urinalysis—Ranges from Newborn/Infant to Adult

Sl. No.	Determination	Age/sex	Normal range
1.	Addis count Leukocytes Erythrocytes casts		< 10 < 5 Occasional hyaline
2.	Colony count, colonies/ml urine	Infant Thereafter	<1000 <10 000
3.	Microscopic leukocytes erythrocytes casts		0–4/HPF Rare/HPF Rare/HPF
4.	Osmolarity	Premature/newborn Thereafter	50–60 mOsm/L 50–1400 > 850 (after fluid restriction)
5.	pH	Newborn/neonate Thereafter	5.0–7.0 4.8–7.8

Contd...

Contd...

Sl. No.	Determination	Age/sex	Normal range
6.	Protein qualitative quantitative		Negative 10–100 mg/day (after strenuous exercise)
7.	Specific gravity, random	Newborn	1.001–1.003
		Infant	1.005–1.030
		Thereafter	1.005–1.030 (after fluid restriction)
8.	Sugar, qualitative (including glucose)		Negative
9.	Volume	Newborn/neonate	50–300 ml/day
		Infant	350–550
		Child	500–1000
		Adolescent	700–1400
		Thereafter:	
		Males:	800–2000
		Females:	800–1600

Normal Serologic Reference Values

Sl. No.	Determination	Normal range
1.	Anti-streptolysin O titre	
	Preschool	<1:85
	School ages and adults	<1:170
	Older adults	<1:85

Contd...

Contd...

Sl. No.	Determination	Normal range
2.	Antihyaluronidase	<1:256
3.	Antinuclear antibody	<1:40
4.	C-reactive protein	Negative
5.	C_3	70–176 mg/dl
6.	C_4	16–45 mg/dl
7.	Carcinoembryonic antigen (CEA)	< 2.5 ng/ml
8.	Febrile agglutinins	<1:80 or four fold rise in titre
9.	Mononucleosis screen	Negative
10.	Proteus OX-19 agglutinins	<1:80 or four fold rise in titre
11.	Rheumatoid latex titre	1:80–1:160 Doubtful 1:40 Negative
12.	Tularemia agglutinins	<1:80 or four fold rise in titre
13.	Waaler-Rose titer	1:10 Negative 1:20–1:40 Doubtful >1:80 Positive
14.	Complement fixation tests should be negative or <1:8	

    Brucellosis

    Cytomegalic inclusion disease

    Eastern and western equine encephalitis

    Epidemic typhus

    Influenza type A

Contd...

Contd...

Sl. No.	Determination
	Influenza type B
	Lymphocytic choriomeningitis
	Lymphogranuloma venereum
	Mumps
	Psittacosis
	Q fever (American)
	Rickettsial pox
	Rocky mountain spotted fever
	St. Louis encephalitis
	Toxoplasmosis
	Tularemia

Chapter 9
Profile of Laboratory Tests According to Body Systems

CARDIOVASCULAR SYSTEM

Cardiac Enzymes

Determination	Normal ranges	
	Conventional units	SI units
Aspartate aminotransferase (AST)	**Males:** 10–40 U/L	0.17–0.68 µkat/L
	Females: 8–35 U/L	0.14–0.60 µkat/L
Creatine phosphokinase (CPK)	**Males:** 50–325 mU/ml	50–325 U/L
	Females: 50–250 mU/ml	50–250 U/L
Creatine kinase, isoenzyme		
CK-MB	0% of total CK	
CK-MM	5–70% of total CK	
Lactic dehydrogenase (LDH)	90–176 mU/ml	90–176 U/L
LDH isoenzymes		
LDH 1	22–36%	0.2–0.36
LDH 2	35–46%	0.35–0.46

Contd...

Contd...

	Normal ranges	
Determination	Conventional units	SI units
LDH 3	13–26%	0.13–0.26
LDH 4	3–10%	0.03–0.10
LDH 5	2–12%	0.02–0.12
Alpha–hydroxybutyrate dehydrogenase (HBDH)	70–300 U/L	
Troponin (contractile protein found only in cardiac muscle)	Elevated in myocardial injury	

Lipids

	Normal ranges	
Determination	Conventional units	SI units
Total lipoprotein	400–800 mg/dl	4–8 gm/L
Lipoprotein electrophoresis: High density lipoprotein (HDL)	20–48 mg/dl	0.51–1.24 mmol/L
Low density lipoprotein (LDL)	38–40 mg/dl	0.98–1.04 mmol/L
Very low density lipoprotein (VLDL)	3–32 mg/dl	–
Cholesterol	150–200 mg/dl	3.9–5.2 mmol/L
Triglycerides	100–200 mg/dl	1.13–3.8 mmol/L
Phospholipids	125–300 mg/dl	1.25–3 gm/L
Free fatty acids	8–25 mg/dl	0.3–0.90 mmol/L

Electrolyte Panel

Determination	Normal ranges	
	Conventional units	SI units
Potassium	3.5–5.0 mEq/L	3.5–5.0 mmol/L
Sodium	135–145 mEq/L	135–145 mmol/L
Chloride	95–105 mEq/L	97–105 mmol/L
Bicarbonate		
• Peripheral vein	19–25 mEq/L	19–25 mmol/L
• Arterial sample	22–26 mEql/L	22–26 mEq/L
Calcium	9–11 mg/dl 4.5–5.5 mEq/L	2.25–2.75 mmol/L
Phosphorus	2.5–4.5 mg/dl	0.8–1.45 mmol/L
Magnesium	1.3–2.3 mg/dl	0.62–0.95 mmol/L

Coagulation

Determination	Normal ranges (Conventional units)
Prothrombin time (PT)	9.5–12 secs
Activated partial thromboplastin time (aPTT)	20–25 secs lower limit 32–39 secs upper limit
International normalized ratio (INR) In treatment	1 2.5–3 in AF, DVT, pulmonary embolism 2.5–3.5 for therapy in prosthetic heart valves
Lee–White coagulation time (LWCT)	4–8 minutes

Drug Levels

Determination	Therapeutic levels	Toxic levels
Digoxin	0.5–2 ng/ml	> 2.5 ng/ml
Digitoxin	10–25 ng/ml	30 ng/ml
Diltiazem	50–200 ng/ml	> 200 ng/ml
Nifedipine	5–10 mg	90 mg
Verapamil	5–10 mg/kg	>15 mg/kg
Propanolol	50–100 ng/ml	> 100 ng/ml

Pericardial Fluid

Determination	Normal ranges
Cytologic examination	No abnormal cells
RBC count	None normally present
WBC count	<1000/mm^3
Glucose	80–100 mg/dl
Microbiologic examination	No organisms present

Miscellaneous

	Normal ranges	
Determination	Conventional units	SI units
Erythrocyte sedimentation rate (ESR)	**Males** < 50 yrs: < 15 mm/hr >50 yrs: < 20 mm/hr	**Males** < 50 yrs: < 15 mm/hr >50 yrs: < 20 mm/hr

Contd...

Contd...

Determination	Normal ranges	
	Conventional units	**SI units**
	Females	**Females**
	<50 yrs: < 25 mm/hr	<50 yrs: < 25 mm/hr
	>50 yrs: < 30 mm/hr	>50 yrs: < 30 mm/hr
Leukocyte count	4,500–11,000/cu.mm	$4.5–11 \times 10^9$/L
• Neutrophils	45–73%	Number fraction 0.45–0.73
• Eosinophils	0–4%	0.00–0.04
• Basophils	0–1%	0.00–0.01
• Lymphocytes	20–40%	0.20–0.40
• Monocytes	2–8%	0.02–0.08
Erythrocyte count	**Males:** 4,600,000–6,200,000/cu.mm	$4.6–6.2 \times 10^{12}$/L
	Females: 4,200,000–5,400,000/cu.mm	$4.2–5.4 \times 10^{12}$/L
Platelet count	1,50,000–4,50,000/cu.mm	$0.15–0.45 \times 10^{12}$/L
Hemoglobin	**Males:** 13–18 gm/dl	2.02–2.79 mmol/L
	Females: 12–16 gm/dl	1.86–2.48 mmol/L
Hematocrit	**Males:** 42–52%	Volume fraction: 0.42–0.52
	Females: 35–47%	Volume fraction: 0.35–47
Glucose	**Fasting:** 60–110 mg/dl	3.3–6.05 mmol/L
	Postprandial 2 hr: 65–140 mg/dl	3.58–7.7 mmol/L

Contd...

Contd...

	Normal ranges	
Determination	Conventional units	SI units
Blood gases		
pH	7.35–7.45	
pCO_2	35–45 mm Hg	
pO_2	75–100 mm Hg	

PULMONARY SYSTEM

Arterial Blood Gases

Determination	Normal ranges
pH	7.35–7.45
pCO_2	35–45 mm Hg
pO_2	75–100 mm Hg
HCO_3	22–26 mEq/L
BE	+ 1 to –2

Sputum

Determination	Normal ranges
Gram stain	Normal sputum contains polymorphonuclear leukocytes, alveolar macrophages and a few squamous epithelial cells
Acid-fast bacilli (AFB) culture and sensitivity	Negative for AFB

Contd...

Contd...

Determination	Normal ranges
Culture and sensitivity	Normal respiratory flora includes Moraxella catarrhalis, *Candida albicans*, diphtheroids, alpha-hemolytic streptococci and some staphylococci

Cytologic examination negative for abnormal cells, Curschmann's spirals, fungi, ova and parasites.

Pleural Fluid

Determination	Normal ranges
Microbiologic examination (culture and sensitivity, Gram stain)	No organisms present
Cytologic examination	No abnormal cells
Lactic dehydrogenase (LDH)	71–207 IU/L
White blood cells (WBC)	0–<1000/m³, consisting mainly of lymphocytes
Red blood cells (RBC)	0–<1000/mm³
pH	7.37–7.43 (usually above 7.40)
Protein	3.0 gm/dl
Immunoglobulins	
Glucose	
Complement	Parallels serum levels
Carcinoembryonic antigen (CEA)	
Cholesterol	
Triglycerides	

Drug Levels

Determination	Therapeutic level	Toxic level
Theophylline therapeutic regimen	10–18 µg/ml	> 20 µg/ml

Miscellaneous

Determination	Normal ranges
Alpha-1 antitrypsin	80–213 mg/dl
White blood cells (WBC)	4,500–11,000/cu.mm

NEUROLOGICAL SYSTEM

CSF Fluid

Determination	Normal ranges
Color	Clear
Pressure	75–200 mm H_2O (average 120 mm H_2O)
Protein	
Lumbar	15–45 mg/dl
Cisternal	15–25 mg/dl
Ventricular	5–15 mg/dl
Cell count	0–5 mononuclear cells/cu.mm
Glucose	50–75 mg/dl
Lactic dehydrogenase	One tenth that of serum
Chloride	100–130 mEq/L

Contd...

Contd...

Determination	Normal ranges
Urea	10–15 mg/dl
Lactic acid	< 24 mg/dl
Glutamine	6–15 mg/dl
Microbiologic examination (C/S and Gram stain)	Organism not normally present in CSF
Cytologic examination	No abnormal cells

Drug Levels

Determination	Therapeutic level	Toxic level
Anticonvulsants: Phenobarbital	10 µg/ml	> 55 µg/ml
Phenytoin	10–20 µg/ml	>20 µg/ml
Sodium valproate	50–100 µg/ml	> 100 µg/ml

Miscellaneous

	Normal ranges	
Determination	Conventional units	SI units
Electrolytes		
♦ Potassium	3.5–5.0 mEq/L	3.5–5.0 mmol/L
♦ Sodium	135–145 mEq/L	135–145 mmol/L
♦ Chloride	95–105 mEq/L	97–105 mmol/L

Contd...

Contd...

Determination	Normal ranges	
	Conventional units	SI units
Bicarbonate		
• Peripheral vein	19–25 mEq/L	19–25 mmol/L
• Arterial sample	22–26 mEq/L	22–26 mEq/L
Calcium	9–11 mg/dl 4.5–5.5 mEq/L	2.25–2.75 mmol/L
Phosphorus	2.5–4.5 mg/dl	0.8–1.45 mmol/L
Magnesium	1.3–2.3 mg/dl	0.62–0.95 mmol/L
Glucose	**Fasting**: 60–110 mg/dl	3.3–6.05 mmol/L
	Postprandial 2 hr: 65–140 mg/dl	3.58–7.7 mmol/L
Alcohol	500 mg/kg (toxic dose)	
Blood urea	10–20 mg/dl nitrogen (BUN)	3.6–7.2 mmol/L
Creatinine	0.7–1.4 mg/dl	62–124 µmol/L

Arterial Blood Gases

Determination	Normal ranges
pH	7.35–7.45
pCO_2	35–45 mm Hg
pO_2	75–100 mm Hg
HCO_3	22–26 mEq/L
BE	+1 to –2

HEMATOLOGICAL SYSTEM

Blood Cell Counts

Determination	Normal ranges	
	Conventional units	SI units
White blood cells (WBC)	4,500–11,000/cu.mm	$4.5-11 \times 10^9/L$
		Number fraction
• Neutrophils	40-73%	0.45–0.73
• Eosinophils	0–4%	0.00–0.04
• Basophils	0–1%	0.00–0.01
• Lymphocytes	20–40%	0.20–0.40
• Monocytes	2–8%	0.02–0.08
Red blood cells (RBC)	**Males:** 4,600,000–6,200,000/cu.mm	$4.6-6.2 \times 10^{12}/L$
	Females: 4,200,000–5,400,000/cu.mm	$4.2-5.4 \times 10^{12}/L$
Platelets	1,50,000–4,50,000/cu.mm	$0.15-0.45 \times 10^{12}/L$
Hemoglobin	**Males:** 13–18 gm/dl	2.02–2.79 mmol/L
	Females: 12–16 gm/dl	1.86–2.48 mmol/L
Hematocrit	**Males:** 42–52%	Volume fraction: 0.42–0.52
	Females: 35–47%	Volume fraction: 0.35–47

Contd...

Contd...

	Normal ranges	
Determination	**Conventional units**	**SI units**

RDW–red cell distribution with width

Erythrocyte indices

- Mean corpuscular volume (MCV)   84–96 cu μm   84–96 femtolitre
- Mean corpuscular Hb (MCH)   28–33 μμg/cell   28–33 picogram
- Mean corpuscular Hb concentration (MCHC)   33–35%   Conc. fraction 0.33–0.35
- Reticulocytes   0.5–1.5% of red cells   Number fraction 0.005–0.015

Blood Cell Types

	Normal ranges	
Determination	**Conventional units**	**SI units**
Hb electrophoresis	95–97%	<0.95
Hgb A	2–3%	0.02–0.03
Hgb A2	>1%	>0.01
Hgb F	2% or 0.06–0.24	
methemoglobin (Hgb M)	g/dl minute amounts	
Sulfhemoglobin	0–2.3%	
Carboxyhemoglobin	4–5% in smokers	

Determination	
Blood typing and cross matching	A, B, O, AB and D antigen is present on red cells of 85% of whites, and higher percentage in blacks, Native Americans and Asians |//

Sickle cell screening Negative

Coagulation Profile

Determination	Normal ranges
Prothrombin time (PT)	9.5–12 secs
Activated partial thromboplastin time (aPTT)	20–25 secs lower limit 32–39 secs upper limit
International normalized ratio (INR) In treatment	1 2.5–3 in AF, DVT, pulmonary embolism 2.5–3.5 for therapy in prosthetic heart valves
Lee–White coagulation time (LWCT)	4–8 minutes
Bleeding time (BT)	1.5–9.5 min
Platelet aggregation	Visible in less than 5 minutes
Clot retraction time	A normal clot is separated from the test tube and incubated at 37°C, shrinks to half its original size within 1 hour. The result is firm, cylindrical fibrin clot that contains all red blood cells and is sharply demarcated from the clear serum

Profile of Laboratory Tests According to Body Systems

Determination	Normal ranges
Capillary fragility	Fewer than 10 petechiae, in a 2-inch circle is considered normal
Thrombin clotting time (TCT)	10–15 seconds
Prothrombin consumption time (PCT)	15–20 seconds

Factor assays

Extrinsic pathway
Factor II 70–130 mg/dl
Factor V 70–130 mg/dl
Factor VII 70–150 mg/dl
Factor X 70–130 mg/dl

Intrinsic pathway
Factor VIII 50–200 mg/dl
Factor IX 70–130 mg/dl
Factor XII 70–130 mg/dl

Common pathway Factor XIII	Dissolution of a formed clot within 24 hours
Plasma fibrinogen	150–450 mg/dl
Fibrin split products (FSP)	2–10 µg/ml
Euglobulinlysis	Lysis in 2–6 hours
D-dimmer (measures amount of fragments of fibrin when lysed)	**Qualitative:** No D-dimmer fragments present **Quantitative:** < 0.25 mg/L

Iron Deficiency

	Normal ranges	
Determination	Conventional units	SI units
Iron	50–160 µg/dl	9–29 µmol/L
Total iron binding capacity (TIBC)	IBC: 250–350 µg/dl	45–63 µmol/L
	TIBC: 250–475 µg/dl	45–85 µmol/L
	% saturation: 20–50	Fraction of TIBC 0.2–0.5

Hemolysis

Determination	Normal ranges
RBC enzymes:	
Glucose 6 phosphate dehydrogenase	4.3–11.8 IU/G Hgb
Haptoglobin	30–160 mg/dl
Indirect Coombs test	Negative (no agglutination)
Bilirubin	**Total:** 0.3–1 mg/dl **Direct:** 0.1–0.4 mg/dl **Indirect:** 0.1–0.4 mg/dl

Miscellaneous

Determination	Normal ranges
Erythrocyte osmotic fragility	**Immediate test:** Hemolysis begins at 0.50 NaCl; complete at 0.30 NaCl **24-hour incubation:** Hemolysis begins at 0.70 NaCl; complete at 0.40–0.15 NaCl

Contd...

Contd...

Determination	Normal ranges
Erythrocyte sedimentation rate (ESR)	**Males** < 50 yrs: < 15 mm/hr >50 yrs: < 20 mm/hr **Females** <50 yrs: < 25 mm/hr >50 yrs: < 30 mm/hr
WBC enzymes: Leukocyte alkaline phosphates (LAP)	13–130 U
Periodic Acid-Schiff (PAS) stain	Granulocytes–positive Granulocytic precursors–negative Erythrocytes–negative Erythrocytic precursors–negative
Tartarate–resistant acid phosphates (TRAP)	Activity absent
T-lymphocytes	60–80% of circulating lymphocytes
B-lymphocytes	10–20% of circulating lymphocytes
Immunoglobulin assay	(in SI Units)
IgG	8–18 gm/L
IgA	1–4 gm/L
IgM	0.55–1.50 gm/L
IgD	0.005–0.03 gm/L
IgE	0–430 µg/L

ENDOCRINE SYSTEM

Thyroid Tests

Determination	Normal ranges	
	Conventional units	*SI units*
Calcitonin	Basal: <19 pg/ml	19 ng/L
	Stimulation test:	
	Males: < 350 pg/ml	< 350 ng/L
	Females: < 100 pg/ml	< 100 ng/L
Thyroid stimulating imunoglobulins (TSI)	**Males:** < 0.155 ng/ml	< 0.155 μgm/L
	Females: < 0.105 ng/ml	< 0.105 μ/L
Thyroxine binding globulin (TBG)	10–26 μg/dl	100–260 μg/L
Triiodothyronine (T3)	70–204 ng/dl	1.08–3.14 nmol/L
T_3 uptake	24–34%	Relative uptake fraction: 0.24–0.34
Thyroxine (T_4)	5–11 μg/dl	65–138 nmol/L
Free T_4 index	0.9–2.3 ng/dl	10–30 nmol/L
Thyroid stimulating hormone	< 10 μ IU/ml	< 10 mU/L
Free T_3	0.2–0.6 ng/dl	0.003–0.009 nmol/L
Reverse T_3	38–44 ng/dl	0.58–0.67 nmol/L

Parathyroid Tests

	Normal ranges	
Determination	Conventional units	SI units
Parathyroid hormone (PTH)	10–65 pg/ml	10–65 ng/L
Calcium	8.6–10.2 mg/dl	2.15–2.55 mmol/L
Phosphorus	2.5–4.5 mg/dl	0.8–1.45 mmol/L

Pituitary Tests

	Normal ranges	
Determination	Conventional units	SI units
Growth hormone (GH) RIA	**Males:** 0–4 ng/ml **Females:** 0–18 ng/ml	0.4 µg/L 0–18 µg/L
Growth suppression	< 3 ng/ml	< 3 µg/L
Growth hormone stimulation test	**Males:** > 10 ng/ml **Females:** > 15 ng/ml	>10 µg/L >15 µg/L
Prolactin	**Males:** 1–20 ng/ml **Females:** Non-lactating: 1–25 ng/ml Menopausal: 1–20 ng/ml	 1–25 µg/L 1–20 µg/L
Adrenocorticotropic hormone (ACTH)		
Bioscience Laboratories	< 80 pg/ml at 8 am	< 17.6 pmol/L
Mayo clinic	< 120 pg/ml at 6–8 am	< 26.4 pmol/L
Thyroid stimulating hormone (TSH)	< 10 uIU/ml	< 10 mU/L

Contd...

Contd...

Determination	
TSH stimulation test	TSH levels rise within 15–30 mts of thyrotropin releasing hormone (TRH) administration, peak at 2.5 to 4 times normal and return to baseline levels within 24 hrs. Thyroid hormone (T_3 and T_4) which should be increased by 50–70% occurs in 1 to 4 hours.

	Normal ranges	
Determination	*Conventional units*	*SI units*
Follicular stimulating hormone (FSH)	**Males:** 10–15 mIU/ml	5–10 IU/L
	Females: Menstruation	
	Early in cycle: 5–25 mIU/ml	10–15 IU/L
	Midcycle: 20–30 mIU/ml	5–25 IU/L
	Luteal phase: 5–25 mIU/ml	20–30 IU/L
	Menopausal: 40–250 mIU/ml	40–250 IU/L
Luteinizing hormone (LH)	**Males:** 1.5–9.3 mU/ml	1.5–9.3 U/L
	Females:	
RIA	Follicular phase: 1.9–12.5 mU/ml	1.9–12.5 U/L
	Midcycle: 8.7–76.3 mU/ml	8.7–76.3 U/L
Antidiuretic hormone (ADH)	2.3–3.1 pg/ml	2.3–3.1 ng/L

Adrenal Tests

Determination	Normal ranges	
	Conventional units	**SI units**
Cortisol–RIA	8 am: 5–25 µg/dl 4 pm: 3–16 µg/dl	138–690 nmol/L 83–442 nmol/L
Adrenocorticotropic hormone (ACTH)–RIA	< 50 pg/ml	< 50 ng/ml
Cortisol–ACTH challenge	Usual response is an increase in plasma cortisol levels of 7–18 µg/dl over baseline levels within 1 hour of administration of ACTH. Lack of response indicated adrenal insufficiency	
Aldosterone (Plasma)–RIA	**Supine:** 3–10 ng/d **Upright:** 5–30 ng/dl **Adrenal vein:** 200–800 ng/dl	0.08–0.30 nmol/L 0.14–0.90 nmol/L 5.54–22.16 nmol/L
Aldosterone challenge	**Supine:** 3–9 ng/dl **Upright:** 5–30 ng/dl	0.08–0.30 nmol/L 0.14–0.80 nmol/L
Catecholamines (plasma) RIA		
Epinephrine	< 100 pg/ml	< 540 pmol/L
Norepinephrine	< 400 pg/ml	< 2360 pmol/L
Dopamine	< 143 pg/ml	< 935 pmol/L
Urinary hormones: Cortisol	20–90 µg/24 hrs	55.2–248.4 nmol/day
Aldosterone	**With normal salt diet** **Normal:** 4–20 µg/24 hrs **Renovascular:** 10–40 µg/24 hrs **Tumor:** 20–100 µg/24 hrs	11.1–55.5 nmol 27.7–111 nmol/24 hrs 55.4–277 nmol/24 hrs

Contd...

Contd...

Determination	Normal ranges	
	Conventional units	SI units
17-hydroxycorticosteroids (17-OHCS)	2 to 8 mg/24 hrs	5.5–27.5 µmol/day
17-ketogenic steroids (17- KGS)	**Males:** 5–23 mg/24 hrs	17–80 µmol/day
	Females: 3–15 mg/24 hrs	10–52 µmol/day
Pregnanetriol	< 3.5 mg/24 hrs	< 10.4 µmol/day
Vanillylmandelic acid (VMA)	0.7–6.8 mg/24 hrs	3–34 µmol/day

Pancreas Tests

Determination	Normal ranges	
	Conventional units	SI unit
Glucose	**Fasting:** 60–110 mg/dl	3.3–6.05 mmol/L
	Postprandial 2 hr: 65–140 mg/dl	3.58–7.7 mmol/L
Glucose tolerance test-Oral test (OGTT)	30 mts: < 150 mg/dl 1 hr: < 160 mg/dl 2 hrs: < 115 mg/dl 3 hrs: Same as fasting level	
IV test (IVGTT)	Same as OGTT, except for blood glucose level at ½ hr interval may be 300–400 mg/dl	
2 hrs (Postprandial blood sugar) PPBS	< 140 mg/dl	7.7 mmol/L
Ketones (urine)	Negative	

Contd...

Contd...

Determination	Normal ranges	
	Conventional units	*SI unit*
Glycohemoglobin (GHB, hemoglobin A 1c, HbA1)	Non-diabetics and diabetics with good control 4.4–6.4% of hemoglobin	
Blood urea nitrogen (BUN)	10–20 mg/dl	3.6–7.2 mmol/L
Creatinine	0.7–1.4 mg/dl	62–124 µmol/L
Tolbutamide tolerance	Decrease in serum glucose in 5–10 mts of administration of drug. Lowest glucose level occurs in 20–30 mts to half of client's fasting level. Returns to pretest value in 1–3 hrs.	
Insulin	Fasting: 8.0–15.0 µU/ml After 100 gm of glucose: 1/2 hr: 25–231 µU/ml 1 hr: 18–276 µU/ml 2 hrs: 16–166 µU/ml 3 hrs: 4–38 µU/ml	55–104 pmol/L 173–1604 pmol/ 125–1916 pmol/ 111–1152 pmol/L 27–263 pmol/L
Amylase	60–160 somogyi U/dl	111–296 U/L
Lipids	400–800 mg/dl	4–8 gm/L
Aldolase	3–8 Sibley–Lehninger U/dl at 37°C	22–59 mU/L at 37°C
Potassium	3.5–5.0 mEq/L	3.5–5.0 mmol/L
Sodium	135–145 mEq/L	135–145 mmol/L
Glucagons	50–200 pg/ml	50–200 ng/L
C-peptide	0.9–4.2 ng/ml	0.30–1.39 nmol/L

RENAL AND UROLOGIC SYSTEM

Blood Tests

Determination	Normal ranges	
	Conventional units	*SI units*
Blood urea nitrogen (BUN)	10–20 mg/dl	3.6–7.2 mmol/L
Creatinine	0.7–1.4 mg/dl	62–124 µmol/L
Osmolality	275–300 mOsm/kg	275–300 mmol/L
Protein–total	6–8 gm/dl	60–80 gm/L
Albumin	4–5.5 gm/dl	40–55 gm/L
Globulin	1.7–3.3 gm/dl	17–33 gm/L
Ammonia (plasma)	15–45 µg/dl	11–32 µmol/L
Uric acid	2.5–8 mg/dl	0.15–0 mmol/L
Renin (plasma) RLA	**Normal diet**	
	Supine: 0.3–1.9 ng/ml/hr	0.08–0.52 ng/L/S
	Upright: 0.6–3.6 ng/ml/hr	0.16–1.00 µg/L/S
	Low salt diet	
	Supine: 0.9–4.5 ng/ml/hr	0.25–1.25 µg/L/S
	Upright: 4.1–9.1 ng/ml/hr	1.13–2.53 µg/L/S
Aldosterone (plasma) RIA	Supine: 3–10 ng/d	0.08–0.30 nmol/L
	Upright: 5–30 ng/dl	0.14–0.90 nmol/L
	Adrenal vein: 200–800 ng/dl	5.54–22.16 nmol/L

Contd...

Contd...

Determination	Normal ranges	
	Conventional units	*SI units*
Gamma glutamyl transpeptidase (GGTP)	**Males:** 6–37 U/L	0.10–0.63 µkat/L
	Females:	
	< 45 yr: 5–27 U/L	0.08–0.46 µkat/L
	> 45 yr: 6–37 U/L	0.10–0.63 µkat/L
Electrolytes		
Potassium	3.5–5.0 mEq/L	3.5–5.0 mmol/L
Sodium	135–145 mEq/L	135–145 mmol/L
Chloride	95–105 mEq/L	97–105 mmol/L
Bicarbonate		
(peripheral vein)	19–25 mEq/L	19–25 mmol/L
(arterial sample)	22–26 mEql/L	22–26 mEq/L
Calcium	9–11 mg/dl	2.25–2.75 mmol/L
	4.5–5.5 mEq/L	
Phosphorus	2.5–4.5 mg/dl	0.8–1.45 mmol/L
Magnesium	1.3–2.3 mg/dl	0.62–0.95 mmol/L

Urine Tests

Determination	Age/sex	Normal range
Addis count		
• Leukocytes		< 10
• Erythrocytes		< 5
• Casts		Occasional hyaline

Contd...

Contd...

Determination	Age/sex	Normal range
Colony count, colonies/ml urine	Infant	<1000
	Thereafter	<10 000
Microscopic		
• Leukocytes		0–4/HPF
• Erythrocytes		Rare/HPF
• Casts		Rare/HPF
Osmolality	Premature/newborn	50–60 mOSm/L
	Thereafter	50–1400
		> 850 (after fluid restriction)
pH	Newborn/neonate	5.0–7.0
	Thereafter	4.8–7.8
Protein		
Qualitative		Negative
Quantitative		10–100 mg/day (after strenuous exercise)
Specific gravity, random	Newborn/infant	1.001–1.020
	Thereafter	1.001–1.030
		>1.025 (after fluid restriction)
Sugar, qualitative (including glucose)		Negative
Volume	Newborn/neonate	50–300 ml/day
	Infant	350–550 ml/day
	Child	500–1000 ml/day
	Adolescent	700–1400 ml/day

Contd...

Contd...

Determination	Age/sex	Normal range
	Thereafter— **Male:** **Female:**	800–2000 ml/day 800–1600 ml/day

	Normal ranges	
Determination	Conventional units	SI units
Creatinine clearance	Males: 85–125 ml/min Females: 75–115 ml/min	1.41–2.08 ml/s 1.21–1.91 ml/s
Protein	Upto 100 mg/24 hrs	
Complement C_3	70–176 mg/dl	
Complement C_4	16–45 mg/dl	
Tubular function [phenolsulphonphthalein (PSP)]	After 15 min: 25% of dose is excreted After 30 min: 50–60% of dose is excreted After 60 min: 60–70% of dose is excreted After 2 hrs: 70–80% of dose is excreted	
Concentration: Osmolality Specific gravity	250–900 mOsm/kg 1.010–1.025	250–900 mmol/kg
Electrolytes		
Calcium	<150 mg/24 hrs	2.5–6.2 mmol/24 hrs
Phosphorus, inorganic	0.9–1.3 gm/24 hrs	29–42 mmol/24 hrs
Potassium	40–65 mEq/24 hrs	
Sodium	130–200 mEq/24 hrs	
Culture and sensitivity	Negative for pathogenic organisms	

MUSCULOSKELETAL SYSTEM

Muscle/Bone Enzymes

Determination	Normal ranges	
	Conventional units	SI units
Aldolase	3–8 Sibley–Lehninger U/dl at 37°C	22–59 mU/L at 37°C
Alkaline phosphatase (ALP)	Adults: 50–120 UL	50–120 UL
Creatine phosphokinase (CPK)	**Males:** 50–325 mU/ml **Females:** 50–250mU/ml	50–325 U/L 50–250 U/L

Bone Metabolism

Determination	Normal ranges	
	Conventional units	SI units
Calcitonin	**Basal:** <19 pg/ml	19 ng/L
	Stimulation test:	
	Males: <350 pg/ml	< 350 ng/L
	Females: <100 pg/ml	< 100 ng/L
Parathyroid hormone	10–65 pg/ml	10–65 ng/L
Thyroid		
Thyroid stimulating imunoglobulins (TSI)	**Males:** < 0.155 ng/ml **Females:** < 0.105 ng/ml	< 0.155 µg/L < 0.105 µg/L

Contd...

Contd...

Determination	Normal ranges	
	Conventional units	SI units
Thyroxine binding globulin (TBG)	10–26 µg/dl	100–260 µg/L
Triiodothyronine (T_3)	70–204 ng/dl	1.08–3.14 nmol/L
T 3 uptake	24–34%	Relative uptake fraction: 0.24–0.34
Thyroxine (T_4)	5–11 µg/dl	65–138 nmol/L
Free T_4 index	0.9–2.3 ng/dl	10–30 nmol/L
Thyroid stimulating hormone	< 10 µ IU/ml	< 10 mU/L
Free T_3	0.2–0.6 ng/dl	0.003–0.009 nmol/L
Reverse T_3	38–44 ng/dl	0.58–0.67 nmol/L
Thyroid stimulating imunoglobulins (TSI)	**Males:** < 0.155 ng/ml **Females:** <0.105 ng/ml	<0.155 µg/L < 0.105 µg/L
Vitamin D	10–55 ng/ml	25–100 pmol/L

Electrolyte

Determination	Normal ranges	
	Conventional units	SI units
Calcium	8.6–10.2 mg/dl	2.15–2.55 mmol/L

Joint Tests

Determination	Normal ranges
Rheumatoid factor (RF)	Negative or < 40 IU/ml
Erythrocyte sedimentation rate (ESR)	**Males** < 50 yrs: < 15 mm/hr >50 yrs: < 20 mm/hr **Females** <50 yrs: < 25 mm/hr >50 yrs: < 30 mm/hr
Antistreptolysin O titer	
Preschool	<1:85
School ages and adults	<1:170
Older adults	<1:85
Immunoglobulin assay	**(in SI Units)**
IgG	8–18 gm/L
IgA	1–4 gm/L
IgM	0.55–1.50 gm/L
IgD	0.005–0.03 gm/L
IgE	0–430 µg/L
Complement C_3	70–176 mg/dl
Complement C_4	16–45 mg/dl

Synovial Fluid

Determination	Normal ranges
Routine analysis	
Red blood cells (RBC)	< 2000/mm^3
White blood cells (WBC)	< 200/mm^3
Neutrophils	< 25%
Protein	< 3 gm/dl
Glucose	< 40 mg/dl
Crystals	None present
Rheumatoid factor	
Antinuclear antibodies (ANA)	Parallels serum values
Uric acid	
Complements	

Urine

Determination	Normal ranges
Calcium	**Males:** < 275 mg/24 hrs
	Females: < 250 mg/24 hrs

HEPATOBILIARY-GI SYSTEMS

Liver Enzymes

Determination	Normal ranges	
	Conventional units	SI units
Alkaline phosphates (ALP)	Adults: 50–120 UL	50–120 UL
Alanine aminotransferase (ALT/SGPT)	**Males:** 10–40 U/L **Females:** 8–35 U/L	0.17–0.68 µkat/L 0.14–0.60 µkat/L
5 nucleotidase	3.2–11.6 IU/L	3.2–11.6 U/L
Lactic dehydrogense (LDH)	90–176 mU/ml	90–176 U/L
LDH isoenzymes		
Total LDH		
LDH 1	22–36%	0.2–0.36
LDH 2	35–46%	0.35–0.46
LDH 3	13–26%	0.13–0.26
LDH 4	3–10%	0.03–0.10
LDH 5	2–12%	0.02–0.12
Leucine aminopeptidase (LAP)	**Males:** 0.8–2.0 mg/dl	61–152 µmol/L
	Females: 0.75–1.85 mg/dl	57–141 µmol/L
Gamma glutamyl transpeptidase (GGTP)	**Males:** 6–37 U/L	0.10–0.63 µkat/L
	Females:	
	<45 yr: 5–27 U/L	0.08–0.46 µkat/L
	> 45 yr: 6–37 U/L	0.10–0.63 µkat/L

Contd...

Contd...

Determination	Normal ranges	
	Conventional units	SI units
Creatine phosphokinase (CPK)	**Males:** 50–325 mU/ml	50–325 U/L
	Females: 50–250 mU/ml	50–250 U/L

Liver Blood Tests

Determination	Normal ranges	
	Conventional units	SI units
Bilirubin	**Total:** 0.3–1 mg/dl	5–17 µmol/L
	Direct: 0.1–0.4 mg/dl	1.7–3.7 µmol/L
	Indirect: 0.1–0.4 mg/dl	3.4–11.2 µmol/L
Protein–total	6–8 gm/dl	60–80 gm/L
Albumin	4–5.5 gm/dl	40–55 gm/L
Globulin	1.7–3.3 gm/dl	17–33 gm/L
Protein **Electrophoresis**		
Albumin	4.0–5.5 gm/dl	40–55 gm/L
Alpha-1-globuln	0.15–0.25 gm/dl	1.5–2.5 gm/L
Alpha-2–globulin	0.43–0.75 gm/dl	4.3–7.5 gm/L
Beta globulin	0.5–1.0 gm/dl	5–10 gm/L
Gamma globulin	0.6–1.3 gm/dl	6–13 gm/L
Prothrombin time (PT)	9.5–12 secs	
Cholesterol	150–200 mg/dl	3.9–5.2 mmol/L

Contd...

Contd...

Determination	Normal ranges	
	Conventional units	SI units
Ammonia (plasma)	15–45 µg/dl	11–32 µmol/L
Hepatitis B–associated antigen and antibody tests (anti–Hbe, HBeAb, HBeAg)	Negative	

Esophageal and Stomach Tests

Determination	Normal ranges	
	Conventional units	SI units
Electrolyte panel		
Potassium	3.5–5.0 mEq/L	3.5–5.0 mmol/L
Sodium	135–145 mEq/L	135–145 mmol/L
Chloride	95–105 mEq/L	97–105 mmol/L
Bicarbonate		
(Peripheral vein)	19–25 mEq/L	19–25 mmol/L
(Arterial sample)	22–26 mEql/L	22–26 mEq/L
Calcium	9–11 mg/dl	2.25–2.75 mmol/L
Phosphorus	2.5–4.5 mg/dl	0.8–1.45 mmol/L
Magnesium	1.3–2.3 mg/dl	0.62–0.95 mmol/L
Gastrin	**Fasting:** 50–150 pg/ml **Postprandial:** 80–170 pg/ml	50–150 ng/L 80–170 ng/L

Gastric Analysis

Determination	Normal ranges
Macroscopic analysis:	
Volume	20–100 ml
Color	Pale gray, translucent
Mucus	Present such that sample is slightly viscous
Blood	Negative
pH	< 2.0
Microscopic analysis:	
Red blood cells	Negative to a few
White blood cells	Negative to a few
Epithelial cells	Few
Bacteria	Absent to few
Yeats	Absent to few
Parasites	Absent
Abnormal	Absent

Small and Large Intestine Tests

Determination	Normal ranges
Carotene	50–300 µg/dl
Carcinoembryonic antigen (CEA)–RLK	0–2.5 µg/L (non-smoker) 0–5 µg/L (smoker)
D-xylose absorption (serum)	At 2 hrs: 30–52 mg/dl
Lactose tolerance test	20–50 mg/dl rise from fasting blood glucose without abdominal symptoms of cramps and diarrhea. Lactose intolerance: < 20 mg/dl of glucose rise from fasting blood glucose with abdominal cramps and diarrhea

Duodenal Contents

Determination	Normal ranges
Macroscopic analysis:	
Volume	20 ml
Color	Pearl gray, translucent
Blood	Negative
pH	8.0–8.5
Bicarbonate	145 mEq/L
Microscopic analysis:	
Red blood cells	Negative
White blood cells	Few
Epithelial cells	Few
Bacteria	Negative
Parasites	Negative

Peritoneal Fluid Analysis

Determination	Normal ranges
Red blood cells	<100,000/mm^3
White blood cells	< 300/mm^3 (undiluted fluid) < 500/mm^3 (lavage fluid)
Neutrophils	<25%
Absolute granulocyte count	< 250/mm^3

Contd...

Contd...

Determination	Normal ranges
Gram stain and culture	No organisms present
AFB smear and culture	No AFB present
Cytologic examination	No abnormal cells present
Glucose	
Amylase	
Ammonia	Parallels serum levels
Alkaline phosphatase	
Creatinine	
Urea	
Carcinoembryonic antigen (CEA)	

Fecal Analysis

Determination	Normal ranges
Occult blood	Negative (0.5–2 ml/day)
Fat	< 5 gm/24 hr
Culture	Normal flora
Trypsin	Positive (+ 2 to 4+)
Urobilinogen	**Random sample:** Negative **24-hr collection:** 40–200 mg/24 hrs
Bile	Negative

REPRODUCTIVE SYSTEM

Female Blood Tests

Determination	Normal ranges	
	Conventional units	SI units
Prolactin–RIA	4–30 ng/ml	4–30 µg/ml
Estrogens, total RIA	**Female:** Cycle days	
	Day 1–10: 61–394 pg/ml	61–394 ng/L
	Day 11–20: 122–437 pg/ml	122–437 ng/L
	Day 21–30: 156–350 pg/ml	156–350 ng/L
	Males: 40–115 pg/ml	40–115 ng/L
Follicle stimulating hormone (FSH)–RIA	**Males:** 2–10 mIU/ml	
	Females:	
	Follicular phase: 5–20 mIU/ml	5–20 IU/L
	Peak of middle cycle:	
	12–30 mIU/ml	12–30 IU/L
	Luteinic phase: 5–15 mIU/ml	5–15 IU/L
	Menopausal females:	
	40–200 mIU/ml	40–200 IU/L
Luteinizing hormone–RIA	**Males:** 1.5–9.3 mU/ml	1.5–9.3 U/L
	Females:	
	Follicular phase 1.9–12.5 mU/ml	1.9–12.5 U/L
	Midcycle: 8.7–76.3 mU/ml	8.7–76.3 U/L
Progesterone–RIA	Follicular phase upto 0.8 ng/ml	2.5 nmol/L
	Luteal phase: 10–20 ng/ml	31.8–63.6 nmol/L
	End of cycle: <1 ng/ml	< 3 nmol/L
	Pregnant: Upto 50 ng/ml in 20th wk	Upto 160 nmol/L

Profile of Laboratory Tests According to Body Systems

Urine Tests

	Normal ranges	
Determination	**Conventional units**	**SI units**
Pregnanediol		
Men	< 1.5 mg/24 hr	< 4.7 µmol/d
Nonpregnant women		
Proliferative phase	0.5–1.5 mg/24hr	1.6–4.7 µmol/d
Luteal phase	2–7 mg/24 hr	6.2–22 µmol/d
Postmenopausal women	0.2–1 mg/24 hr	0.6–3.1 µmol/d
Pregnant women		
16 wk	5–21 mg/24 hr	15–65 µmol/d
20 wk	6–26 mg/24 hr	18–81 µmol/d
24 wk	12–32 mg/hr	37–100 µmol/d
28 wk	19–51 mg/24 hr	59–160 µmol/d
32 wk	22–66 mg/24 hr	68–206 µmol/d
36 wk	22–77 mg/hr	40–240 µmol/d
40 wk	23–83 mg/hr	72–197 µmol/d
Estrogen		
Adult men	4–24 µg/24 hr	4–24 µg/d
Nonpregnant women		
Preovulatory phase	5–25 µg/24 hr	5–25 µg/d
Ovulatory phase	24–100 µg/24hr	24–100 µg/d
Luteal phase	12–80 µg/24 hr	12–80 µg/d
Postmenopausal phase	< 10 µg/24 hr	< 10 µg/d

Blood Tests

Determination	Normal ranges	
	Conventional units	SI units
Testosterone		
Men		
< 60 yr	3.9–7.9 ng/ml	13.59–27.41 nmol/L
> 60 yr	1.5–3.1 ng/ml	5.20–10.75 nmol/L
Women		
Menstruating	0.25–0.67 ng/ml	0.87–2.32 nmol/L
Menopause	0.21–0.37 ng/ml	0.72–1.28 nmol/L
Semen analysis		
pH	>7.0	
Volume	0.7–6.5 ml/ejaculate	
Sperm count	40–160 million/ml (20–40 million/ml= borderline normal)	
Sperm motility	> 60% within 3 hr of specimen collection	
Sperm morphology	< 30% abnormal sperm	
Fructose	Present and/or > 150 mg/dL	
Sperm antibodies	Negative for male and female antibodies	
Postcoital test	At least 10 motile sperm per high power microscopic field within 6–8 hr of coitus	
Acid phosphatase	2500 King–Armstrong U/ml	
Chromosomal analysis	Normal karyotype	

Male Urine Tests

Determination	Normal ranges	
	Conventional units	SI units
17-ketosteroids (17-KS)	**Males:** 10–22 mg/24 hrs	10–22 mg/24 hrs
	Females: 6–16 mg/24 hrs	21–55 µmol/24 hrs

Pregnant Female Tests

Determination	Normal ranges	
	Conventional units	SI units
Complete blood count (CBC)		
White blood cells (WBC)	4,500–11,000/cu.mm	$4.5–11 \times 10^9$/L
		Number fraction
Neutrophils	45–73%	0.45–0.73
Eosinophils	0–4%	0.00–0.04
Basophils	0–1%	0.00–0.01
Lymphocytes	20–40%	0.20–0.40
Monocytes	2–8%	0.02–0.08
Red blood cells (RBC)	**Males:** 4,600,000–6,200,000/cu.mm	$4.6–6.2 \times 10^{12}$/L
	Females: 4,200,000–5,400,000/cu.mm	$4.2–5.4 \times 10^{12}$/L

Contd...

Contd...

Determination	Normal ranges	
	Conventional units	SI units
Platelets	1,50,000–4,50,000/cu.mm	0.15–0.45 × 10^{12}/L
ABO typing and cross matching	A, B, O, AB and D antigen is present on red cells of 85% of whites, and higher percentage in blacks, Native Americans and Asians	
Albumin	4–5.5 gm/dl	40–55 gm/L

Syphilis serology:

Rapid plasma reagin (RPR)	Nonreactive: Negative for syphilis	
Venereal disease research laboratory (VDRL)		
Renin (plasma) RLA	**Normal diet** Supine: 0.3–1.9 ng/ml/hr 0.08–0.52 ng/L/S	
	Upright: 0.6–3.6 ng/ml/hr 0.16–1.00 µg/L/S	
	Low salt diet: Supine: 0.9–4.5 ng/ml/hr 0.25–1.25 µg/L/S	
	Upright: 4.1–9.1 ng/ml/hr 1.13–2.53 µg/L/S	

Contd...

Determination	Normal ranges	
	Conventional units	**SI units**
TORCH (Toxoplasmosis, Other infections, Rubella, Cytomegalovirus and Herpes simplex)	*Negative for* Toxoplasmosis Other infections Rubella Cytomegalovirus Herpes simplex	
Human placental lactogen (HPL)		
Men	< 0.5 µg/ml	Not detected
Women		
Nonpregnant	< 0.5 µg/ml	Not detected
Pregnant		
5–27 wks	< 4.6 µg/ml	< 4.6 mg/L
28–31 wks	2.4–6.1 µg/ml	2.4–6.1 mg/L
32–35 wks	3.7–7.7 µg/ml	3.7–7.7 mg/L
36 wks–term	5.0–8.6 µg/ml	5.0–8.6 mg/L
Diabetic at term	10–12 µg/ml	10–12 mg/L
Creatinine phosphokinase (CPK)	**Males:** 50–325 mU/ml	50–325 U/L
	Females: 50–250 mU/ml	50–250 U/L

Contd...

Contd...

Determination	Normal ranges	
	Conventional units	SI units
Human chorionic gonadotropin (HCG)	**Qualitative:** Negative in no pregnant **Quantitative:** **Men:** < 5.0 IU/L **Nonpregnant women:** < 5.0 IU/L **Pregnant women:** 1 wk of gestation: 5–50 IU/L 2 wk of gestation: 50–500 IU/L 3 wk of gestation: 100–10,000 IU/L 4 wk of gestation: 1080–30,000 IU/L 6–8 wk of gestation: 3,500–115,000 IU/L 12 wk of gestation: 12,000–270,000 IU/L 13–16 wk of gestation: upto 200,000 IU/L 17–40 wk of gestation: graded fall to 4000 IU/L	
Progesterone–RIA	**Follicular phase** upto 0.8 ng/ml	2.5 nmol/L
	Luteal phase: 10–20 ng/ml	31.8–63.6 nmol/L
	End of cycle: <1 ng/ml	<3 nmol/L
	Pregnant: upto 50 ng/ml in 20th wk	Upto 160 nmol/L

Determination	Normal ranges	
	Conventional units	SI units
Urinary pregnanediol	**See above**	
Hematology panel for blood cells	**See above**	

Contd...

Contd...

	Normal ranges	
Determination	**Conventional units**	**SI units**
Coagulation	*See earlier chapters*	
Iron, folate	*See earlier chapters*	
Routine urinalysis	*See earlier chapters*	
Amniotic fluid analysis for lecithin: sphingomyelin ratio (L: S ratio)	< 1.6: 1 before 35 weeks > 2.0: 1 at term	
Chromosomal analysis	Normal karyotype	
Creatinine	1.8–4.0 mg/dl at term	
Phosphatidylglycerol (PG)	Present at approximately 36 weeks	
Alpha fetoprotein	13–41 µg/ml at 13–14 weeks 0.2–3.0 µg/ml at term	

IMMUNE AND AUTOIMMUNE CONDITIONS

Determination	Normal ranges
T and B lymphocyte assay:	
T lymphocytes	60–80% of circulating lymphocytes
B lymphocytes	10–20% of circulating lymphocytes
Null cells	5–20% of circulating lymphocytes
Helper T lymphocytes	50–65% of circulating lymphocytes

Contd...

Contd...

Determination	Normal ranges
Suppressor T lymphocytes	20–35% of circulating lymphocytes
Ratio of helper to suppressor T lymphocyte	2:1
Immunoblast transformation: • Nonimmunee transformation tests • Antigen-specific transformation tests • Mixed lymphocyte culture	• A stimulation index of greater than 10 indicates immunocompetence • A stimulation index of greater 3 indicates prior exposure to the antigen • Nonresponsiveness indicates good histocompatibility
Immunoglobulin assay	(in SI Units)
IgG	8–18 gm/L
IgA	1–4 gm/L
IgM	0.55–1.50 gm/L
IgD	0.005–0.03 gm/L
IgE	0–430 µg/L
Antinuclear antibodies	Negative, <1:40
Uric acid	2.5–8 mg/dl
Rheumatoid factor (RF)	Negative or < 40 IU/ml

Contd...

Contd...

Determination	Normal ranges
Antistreptolysin O titre	
Preschool	<1:85
School ages and adults	<1:170
Older adults	<1:85
C–reactive protein (CRP)	< 0.8 mg/dl
Protein electrophoresis	
Albumin	3.5–5 gm/dl
Globulin	1.5–3.5 gm/dl
Alpha 1	0.1–0.4 gm/dl
Alpha 2	0.4–1.0 gm/dl
Beta	0.5–1.1 gm/dl
Gamma	0.5–1.7 gm/dl
Lupus erythematosus (LE)	Negative, no LE cells
Complement C_3	70–176 mg/dl
Complement C_4	16–45 mg/dl
ESR	**Males** < 50 yrs: < 15 mm/hr >50 yrs:< 20 mm/hr **Females** <50 yrs: < 25 mm/hr >50 yrs:< 30mm/hr
Human immunodeficiency virus (HIV)	Seronegative–no HIV -1 antibodies found in serum

TUMORS

Tumor Marker Tests

Determination	Normal ranges
Prostate (prostate acid phosphatase (PAP))	0–0.8 U/L
Prostate specific antigen (PSA)	> 40 yr: < 2.0 ng/ml < 40 yr: < 2.8 ng/ml
Thyroid (calcitonin)	**Basal:** <19 pg/ml **Stimulation test:** **Males:** <350 pg/ml **Females:** <100 pg/ml
Liver, testes [alpha fetoprotein (AFP)]	< 30 ng/ml
Human chorionic gonadotropin (hCG))	Negative if not present
Ovary (CA125)	0–35 IU/ml
Breast (CA 15-3)	<35 IU/ml
Pancreas (CA-50)	< 37 IU/ml
Colon (CA 19-9, CA- 50)	< 37 IU/ml
Lymphocytes B and T assay	**See above**

Other Tumor Tests

Tumor markers:
- Oncogenes [DNA sequences by polymerase chain reaction (PCR)]
- Cytology examination for B and T cell gene arrangement
- DNA content of tumor cells
- Vasoactive intestinal peptide (VIP)
- Squamous cell carcinoma (SCC) antigen
- Tissue polypeptide antigen (TPA)
- Neuron specific enolase (NSE) Glycoprotein antigen (DU–PAN–2)

Profile of Laboratory Tests According to Body Systems

Other tests	Conventional units	SI units
Metabolic tests		
Uric acid	2.5–8 mg/dl	0.15–0 mmol/L
Albumin	4–5.5 gm/dl	40–55 gm/L
Cholesterol	150–200 mg/dl	3.9–5.2 mmol/L
Triglycerides	100–200 mg/dl	1.13–3.8 mmol/L
Hematologic tests		
Leukocytes	4,500–11,000/cu.mm	$4.5–11 \times 10^9$/L
Platelets	1,50,000–4,50,000/cu.mm	$0.15–0.45 \times 10^{12}$/L
Endocrine tests		
Antidiuretic hormone (ADH)	2.3–3.1 pg/ml	2.3–3.1 ng/L
Cortisol	8 am: 5–25 µg/dl	138–690 nmol/L
	4 pm: 3–16 µg/dl	83–442 nmol/L
Adrenocorticotropic hormone (ACTH)	< 50 pg/ml < 50 ng/ml	
Isoenzymes: Alkaline phosphatase (ALP)	Adults: 50–120 UL	50–120 UL
Creatine kinase	**Males:** 50–325 mU/ml	50–325 U/L
	Females: 50–250 mU/ml	50–250 U/L
Lactate dehydrogenase (LDH)	90–176 mU/ml	90–176 U/L

Index

Page numbers followed by *f* refer to figure and *t* refer to table.

A

Abdominal paracentesis, indications for 97
Accidental stick, cases of 20
Acetaminophen 42
Acetoacetic acid 61, 74
Acid phosphatase 41
Acid-hematin 52
Acidic urine 54
Acute febrile diseases 52
Acute nephritis 57
Adrenal tests 157
Albuminuria 57
Aldolase 41
Alkaline
　phosphatase 41
　urine 54
　　orange-yellow in 53
Alkaptonuria 52
Alpha antitrypsin 31
Alpha-fetoprotein 31
Amikacin 42
Aminobenzoic acid 71
Aminophylline 47
Amitriptyline 43
Ammonia 31, 96
Amniocentesis 98
Amniotic fluid analysis 98
Amobarbital 43
Amphetamine 43
Amylase 41
Angiotensin 31
　converting enzyme 31
Antidiuretic hormone 156
Antistreptolysin O titer 166, 183
Anuria 58
Anus 87
Arterial blood gases 143, 147
Artery, inadvertent puncture of 21
Arthritis, synovial analysis in 93
Ascaris lumbricoides 104
Ascorbic acid 69

B

B lymphocyte assay 181
Bacillary dysentery, chronic 85
Bayer's multistix strips 76
Bicarbonate 32, 161, 170
Bilirubin 32, 61, 62, 69, 72, 98
Bilirubinuria 52
Blood 63, 70
　cell counts 148
　cell types 149
　collections 21
　　of sample of 5
　sampling system 24
　stops 21
　tests 160, 176

Blot 77f
Body excreta analysis 48
Body fluids 89
  analysis 89
Body systems 138
Bone
  enzymes 164
  metabolism 164
Boric acid 51
Bottle 9
Bowel
  large 87
  small 87
Bromide 43
Bronchial casts 104
Broncholiths 104
Butazolidin 46

C

Caffeine 43
Calcitonin 32
Calcium 33
Captopril 70
Carbamazepine 43
Carbenicillin 43
Carbohydrate, abnormalities of 72
Cardiac enzymes 138
Cardiovascular system 138
Catapres 44
Catecholamines 32, 157
Cells and casts 50
Cerebellar pressure, production of 91
Cerebrospinal fluid 89, 131, 145
Ceruloplasmin 33
Cheesy masses 103
Chloral hydrate 43

Chloramphenicol 43
Chlordiazepoxide 43
Chloride, concentrations of 89
Chlorpromazine 43
Chlorpropamide 43
Cholesterol 33, 96
Chorionic gonadotropin 32
Cimetidine 43
Clonazepam 44
Clonidine 44
Clonopin 44
Clotted specimen 19
Coagulation 140
  profile 150
Cocaine 44
Codeine 44
Colchicine 87
Collection issues 16
Collection tray, instruments for 7t
Complete blood count 177
Conversion tables 25
Coproporphyrins 33
Cough swab method 102
Coumadin 47
Creatinine 99
Cyclic adenosine monophosphate 35

D

Dehydroepiandrosterone sulfate 35
Demerol 44
Deoxy corticosterone 35
Desipramine 44
Diabetes management 79
Diabinese 43
Diarrheal stool 80
Diazepam 44

Digitoxin 44, 141
Digoxin 44, 141
Dilantin 46
Dilaudid 44
Diltiazem 141
Dip 77f
Disulfiram 44
Dittrich's plugs 104
Diurnal rhythm 18
Dopamine 32
Doxepin 44
Drug levels 141, 145, 146
Duodenal contents 172
Dyspnea 97

E

Echinococcus granulosus 104
Ehrlich's reagent 71
Electrolyte 161, 163, 165
   panel 140, 170
Electrophoresis 169
Endocrine
   system 154
   tests 185
Enzyme 41
Eosinophils 101
Epinephrine 32
Erythrocytes 29, 73
Escherichia coli 54
Esophageal test 170
Estrogen 175
Ethanol 44
Ethchlorvynol 44
Ethosuximide 44
Excessive sweating 57

F

Fecal analysis 173
Feces 79
   inspection of 81, 84t
Female blood tests 174
Fetal hemoglobin 30
Fibrinogen 30
Fingerstick collection, performance
      of 15
Foreign bodies 104
Formalin 51

G

Gastric analysis 134, 171
Gastrointestinal systems 168
Gentamicin 45
Globulin 154
Glomerulonephritis, chronic 58
Glucose 62, 69
   concentrations, higher 74
Glutamine, concentrations of 89
Glutethimide 45
Glycosuria 57
Gout 94
Gram 27

H

Haemoglobin 30
Haloperidol 45
Handling bayer reagent strips,
      procedures for 65
Haptoglobin 30
Hematocrit 29
Hematologic tests 185

Hematological system 148
Hematology 29, 105
Hematoma 14
  prevention of 16
  size of 21
Hemoconcentration, prevention of 17
Hemoglobin 73
  concentration 75
Hemoglobinuria 52
Hemolysis 152
  prevention of 16
Hepatobiliary 168
Homogentisic acid 52
Hormone 156
  receptors 36
Hospital setup, list of samples in 5t
Human chorionic gonadotropin 180
Human placental lactogen 179
Hydroxybutyric dehydrogenase 41
Hydroxycorticosteroids 35
Hypochlorite 70
Hypodermic syringe 16
Hyposthenuric 57

I

Ibuprofen 45
Imipramine 45
Immune and autoimmune conditions 181
Immunoblast transformation 182
Immunodiagnostic test 128
Immunoglobulin assay 166, 182
Immunologic stimulus 101
Incomplete collection 20
Indole 85
Indomethacin 87

Indoxyl sulfate 69
Indwelling catheter 17
Inflammatory stimulus 101
Inorganic constituents 49
Inorganic phosphorus 37
International system of units 2, 25
International unit 28
Iron deficiency 152
Isocitrate dehydrogenase 42
Isoenzymes 185
Isoniazid 45

J

Joint tests 166

K

Kanamycin 45
Ketogenic steroids 35
Ketone 63, 70, 72
  bodies 69
Ketosteroids 35

L

Laboratory investigations 105
Laboratory tests, profile of 138
Lactate dehydrogenase 42, 96
Large intestine tests 171
Lead 37
Lecithin 99
Librium 43
Lidocaine 45
Lipase 42
Lipid 139
  metabolism 72
Lithium 45

Litre 25
Liver
    abscess 103
    blood tests 169
    disease 69
    enzymes 168
Lorazepam 45
Lumbar cerebrospinal fluids 89
Lumbar puncture 90, 91
    complications of 91
    indications 90
Lung stones 104
Luteinizing hormone 156

M

Magnesium, concentrations of 89
Male urine tests 177
Malic dehydrogenase 42
Mast cells 101
Melanin 52
Meperidine 44
Meprobamate 45
Metabolic tests 185
Methadone 45
Methaqualone 45
Methemoglobinuria 52
Methotrexate 45
Methsuximide 46
Methyldopa 46
Microbial peroxidase 70
Miscellaneous values 132
Mole 27
Monitoring therapy 4
Morphine 46
Mucus 85
Multiple˙ reagent strips 61

Multistix configurations 78
Multistix˙ urinalysis strips 76, 76f
Muscle 164
Musculoskeletal system 164
Myoglobin 73
Myoglobinuria 52

N

Nalidixic acic 74
Nephritis, chronic 57
Neurological system 145
Nifedipine 141
Nontechnical reasons 19
Norepinephrine 32
Normal serologic reference values 135
Normal sputum 103
Normal urine specimens 72
Normetanephrine 32
Nortriptyline 46

O

Occult blood 88
Oliguria 58, 59
    causes of 57
Ordering laboratory tests, purposes for 4
Organic constituents 49
Osteoarthritis 94
Oxazepam 46

P

Pancreas tests 158
Paragonimus westermani 104
Paraldehyde 46
Parasites 104

Parathyroid tests 155
Patient preparation factors 18
Patient's bill of rights 12
Pediatric phlebotomy 22
Percodan 46
Pericardial fluid 95, 141
Peripheral venous blood, collection of 6
Peritoneal fluid 95
   analysis 172
   parameter 95
pH 63, 70, 99
Phenacetin 46
Phenobarbital 46
Phenol poisoning 52
Phenylbutazone 46
Phenytoin 46
Phlebotomy 9t
   collection tubes for 22
Phosphate 37
Pituitary tests 155
Plasma 30, 108, 157
   cells 101
Platelet count 29
Pleural fluid 92, 144
Polyuria 58, 59
Porphobilinogen 34
Porphyria 52
Potassium 38
Pregnanediol 175
Pregnant female tests 177
Primidone 46
Probabilistic nature 3
Procainamide 46
Progesterone 180
Prolonged tourniquet application 17

Propanolol 141
Propoxyphene 47
Propranolol 47
Protein 38, 63, 71, 162
   error indicators 63
Proteinuria 73
Proteus 54
Pulmonary gangrene 103
Pulmonary system 143
Pus 85
Putrid bronchitis 104
Pyridium 52

Q

Quinidine 47
Quinine 47

R

Rauwolfia derivatives 87
Reagents 64
Rectum 87
Red blood cell
   count 29
   enzymes 152
Refractometre 56
Renal system 160
Reproductive system 174
Reticulocytes 29
Rheumatoid arthritis 94
Routine analysis 98
Rust colored sputum 103

S

Safety and infection control 19
Salicylates 74, 87

Salicylic acid 47
Sample collection
 by technical personnel 5
 by ward sisters 5
 procedure of 6
 trolley 7
Sample tube types 9t
Semen analysis 176
Septic arthritis 94
Serum 108
 separation tube 10
Sinequan 44
Skatole 85
Small intestine tests 171
Smaller collection tubes 23
Sodium 38
 concentrations of 89
Specimen
 collection 66, 101
 hemolysis of 19
 preservation of 51
Sputum 101, 103, 143
 examination 101, 102
Steroids 87
Stomach test 170
Stool
 analysis, normal values in 81, 82t
 collections of sample of 5
 mucus in 86t
Stool examination 79
 blood 86
 causes 87
 odor and ph 85
 specimen collection 80
Strip tests 60, 61
Swabs, collections of sample of 5

Synovial fluid 167
 analysis 93
Syphilis serology 178
System international units 28
Systemic lupus erythematosus 94

T

T lymphocyte assay 181
Tagamet 43
Tegretol 43
Testosterone 38
Theophylline 47
Therapeutic drug 42
 monitoring 18
Thorazine 43
Thymol 51
Thyroid 164
 stimulating
  hormone 154
  imunoglobulins 154
Thyroid tests 154
Thyroxine 154
 binding 154
Tobramycin 47
Toluol 51
Toxic drug 42
Toxocara canis 104
Tracheobronchial secretions 101
Transaminases 42
Transudate 96
Triiodothyronine 154
Troubleshooting guidelines 20
Tuberculosis 103
Tuberculous arthritis 94
Tumor 184
 marker tests 184
 tests 184

U

Ulcerative colitis, chronic 85
Units, symbols of 26*t*
Urea splitting 54
Uric acid 100
Urinalysis 61, 134
Urinary hormones 157
Urinary tract infection 55
Urinary volume 58
Urine 167
   analysis 48
   chemistry 122
   collection of 50
      sample of 5
   composition of 48
   gross examination of 51
   pH 54
   physicochemical characteristics of 48
   sample 72
   specimen 71
   tests 161, 175

Urinometre 56, 56*f*
Urobilinogen 64, 71, 73
Urobilinogenuria 52
Urologic system 160

V

Vacutainer 9*t*
   tubes containing blood, range of 23*f*
Valproic acid 47
Vancomycin 47
Vanillylmandelic acid 40
Vein, palpation of 14
Venipuncture 9*t*, 13
   site selection 13
   procedure of 8
Verapamil 141

W

Warfarin 47
White blood cell 97
   count 29
   enzymes 153

EU GSPR Authorised Reprsentative
Logos Europe, 9 rue Nicolas Poussin
1700, La Rochelle, France
Phone: +33 (0) 6 67 93 73 78
E-mail: contact@logoseurope.eu

www.ingramcontent.com/pod-product-compliance
Ingram Content Group UK Ltd.
Pitfield, Milton Keynes, MK11 3LW, UK
UKHW021829140426
5217IPUK00021B/1341